Dynamics of Strength Training and Conditioning

Gary Moran, Ph.D., M.A., FACSM, is the president of Biomechanical Analysis and Research, the Director of Sports Medicine with Biosports, Inc., Research Associate at Ralph K. Davies Medical Center in San Francisco, former visiting professor at the University of California, Berkeley, and a professor at the University of San Francisco. Dr. Moran has an M.A. in Exercise Physiology from San Diego State University and a Ph.D. in Anatomy and Kinesiology (Biomechanics) from the University of Oregon. Dr. Moran has done extensive research in the sports medicine field and has worked with athletes and teams at the university, post-graduate, Olympic, and professional levels. He was the Director of Research at the Nike Shoe Company and Associate Director of Biomechanics at Shriners Hospital for Crippled Children. Dr. Moran is considered an authority on physical fitness, weight training, and the biomechanics of running, cycling, and the triathlon.

Dr. George McGlynn is professor and Chairman of the Department of Exercise and Sport Science at the University of San Francisco. He received his A.B. and M.A. at Syracuse University and his doctorate at the University of California at Berkeley. He is the author of numerous articles, and received the Liberal Arts' College Merit Award for outstanding teaching and research. In addition, he is the author of the highly successful text *Dynamics of Fitness*. He has served as a fitness consultant for a number of federal and state agencies, and helped to plan and supervise the first cardiac rehabilitation program in the San Francisco Bay area.

Second Edition

Dynamics of Strength Training and Conditioning

Gary T. Moran Ph.D., M.A., FACSM

President, Biomechanical Analysis and Research

University of San Francisco

George McGlynn Ed.D., M.A.

University of San Francisco

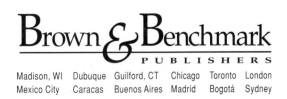

Brown & Benchmark
PUBLISHERS

Madison, WI   Dubuque   Guilford, CT   Chicago   Toronto   London
Mexico City   Caracas   Buenos Aires   Madrid   Bogotá   Sydney

Book Team

Executive Managing Editor *Ed Bartell*
Project Editor *Theresa Grutz*
Production Editor *Patricia A. Schissel*
Proofreading Coordinator *Carrie Barker*
Art Editor *Miriam Hoffman*
Photo Editor *Rose Deluhery*
Production Manager *Beth Kundert*
Production/Imaging and Media Development Manager *Linda Meehan Avenarius*
Production/Costing Manager *Sherry Padden*
Visuals/Design Freelance Specialist *Mary L. Christianson*
Senior Marketing Manager *Pamela S. Cooper*
Copywriter *Sandy Hyde*
Proofreader *Ann Morgan*

Basal Text   10/12 Garamond Light
Display Type   Garamond
Typesetting System   Macintosh/Quark XPress
Paper Stock   50# Restore Cote

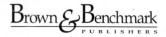

Executive Vice President and General Manager *Bob McLaughlin*
Vice President, Business Manager *Russ Domeyer*
Vice President of Production and New Media Development *Victoria Putman*
National Sales Manager *Phil Rudder*
National Telesales Director *John Finn*

 A Times Mirror Company

The credits section for this book begins on page 159 and is considered an extension of the copyright page.

Cover design by *Kristyn Kalnes*

Cover image by © *Digital Stock*

Copyedited by *John Mulvihill*

Proofread by *Nancy Phan*

Library of Congress Catalog Card Number: 95–83954

ISBN 0–697–12655–2

Printed in the United States of America by Times Mirror Higher Education Group, Inc., 2460 Kerper Boulevard, Dubuque, IA 52001

10 9 8 7 6 5 4 3 2 1

To my wife, Ingeborg, and my son, George.

George McGlynn

To my sister, Deborah Denise Brown, and in memory of my
grandmother, May Sheehan, for their unconditional love.

Gary Moran

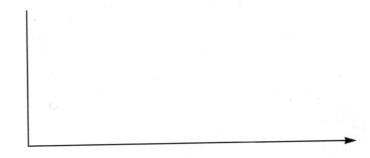

contents

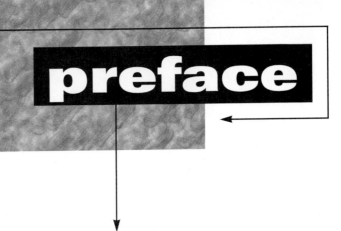

preface

Since the completion of the first edition there have been a number of advances and refinements in the area of muscle strength and endurance. As with the first edition, the purpose of the second edition is to give clarity to this new information by providing a simple, logical, and individualized approach to strength and endurance training. Further, our intent is to enable the reader to distinguish between what is valid and safe from that which is false and dangerous. The book also is intended to be a practical guide for understanding the physiological basis for muscle strength and endurance and the most efficient and effective strength training techniques. The information presented here represents a consensus of presently available scientific evidence.

Approach

This book attempts to bridge the gap between scientific knowledge and the application of that knowledge and also to provide you with the most efficient and up-to-date methods of strength training to insure that your body's adaptations from the training are beneficial and safe. The book also answers basic questions about how to select and prepare for the physical training and how the exercise affects you physically over both short and long periods of exercise.

A sequence of simple tests enables you to evaluate not only your present muscle strength and endurance, but also your cardiorespiratory endurance, body density, and flexibility. The first part of the book describes the benefits of strength training, basic fundamentals and exercises, motivational and mental concentration techniques, and muscle training procedures. Other important areas covered are cardiorespiratory endurance, strength training for women, injuries, nutrition, drugs, flexibility, and an analysis of various strength training equipment.

This text is intended primarily for college classes in physical fitness, strength and weight, circuit training, and body building.

New to This Edition

A number of additions and changes have been made in this new edition. Updated information on the measurement of abdominal strength and flexibility has been added to the chapter on evaluation. A new chapter on flexibility has been added, with an expanded number of flexibility exercises. A pre-exercise screening test (r-PARQ) has been added to the chapter on cardiorespiratory endurance. There are also expanded discussions of plyometrics, periodization, isokinetics, and body building. The chapter on drugs includes new information on fraudulent supplements and an expanded discussion of ergogenic aids and anabolic steroids. A vitamin and mineral chart has been added to the appendix.

Interaction has been increased by the addition of thought-provoking questions throughout the text. Look for the graphic of a notebook and pencil in the margin, identifying each evaluation question.

chapter 1

introduction

Objectives

After studying this chapter you should be able to:

1. Describe some of the misconceptions concerning strength training.
2. Describe the physiological benefits of strength training.
3. Describe the psychological benefits of strength training.
4. Describe the body's adaptation to strength training.
5. Define body building.
6. Define muscle endurance.
7. Define muscle power.
8. Define muscle strength.
9. Define conditioning.
10. Define weight lifting.
11. Define power lifting.
12. Define weight training.

IMPORTANCE OF STRENGTH TRAINING

Little doubt remains today as to the importance of muscular strength and endurance in competitive sports and in the demands of everyday physical activities. Whether you are an athlete looking for increased performance, a sedentary individual dissatisfied with your present lifestyle, or just someone in search of a healthful and satisfying exercise experience, strength training can play a major part in meeting your needs. All that you need is a willingness and determination to take on a new and exciting challenge.

MISCONCEPTIONS

Muscle strength training for many years had been associated with physical fitness. The individual who spent hours in the gym lifting weights had always been considered the model of fitness. We know today, however, that strength training, though essential, is only one aspect of total body fitness. In the past many competitive athletes generally avoided strength training because they thought such training exercises were detrimental to the development and maintenance of certain sports skills. Fears that strength training would bring muscle-boundness, loss of flexibility, and reduced coordination were generally accepted. Current research, however, tells us these concepts are erroneous. Strength training is essential for competitive athletes and also plays a role in determining one's physical fitness level. It is not unusual to see weight lifters engaged in long-distance running and competitive long-distance runners spending more time in weight training. In addition, we now know that resistance training not only leads to increased strength and power but also increases flexibility. The latter benefit puts to rest outdated fears of muscle-boundness.

SUPPLEMENTS

Unsound claims for supplements enter your world daily from radio, television, health clubs, books, magazines, and newspapers. Separating facts from fiction is difficult sometimes even for professionals.

A number of products purported to increase muscle growth, boost energy, increase strength, and reduce body fat are completely fraudulent. Over 2 billion dollars a year are spent on unnecessary vitamins and supplements. Seventy million Americans take vitamin supplements they don't need, and 14 billion dollars are spent on products that amount to pure quackery, from bee pollen to chromium. Herbal remedies, mega doses of vitamins, and mineral therapies are not reliable or effective and may be dangerous to your health.

Many promoters of these ineffective and unproven remedies sincerely believe in the products themselves. In their naivety and enthusiasm they unfortunately pass on the misinformation.

MUSCLE STRENGTH, ENDURANCE, POWER, AND CONDITIONING

The terms strength, muscle endurance, and power are sometimes used interchangeably. However, each of these terms has its own definition. Muscle strength is the amount of force that can be exerted by a muscle group for one movement or repetition. Muscle endurance is the ability of the muscle group to maintain a continuous contraction or repetition over a period of time. Power is simply the product of strength and speed and the ability of the muscle to produce high levels of force in a short period of time. Conditioning is the development of high levels of skeletal muscle strength and endurance, and a high level of cardiorespiratory endurance. This enables one to perform at a high work level for prolonged periods. The muscle system is the foundation of all physical exercise. No matter what activity you participate in, your muscle strength, endurance, and power determine your exercise limits.

In addition, there are other terms that are commonly misused; therefore it seems appropriate to define them before any further discussion.

Weight Lifting is a competitive sport where an individual is judged on the amount of weight that can be lifted relative to weight classification. The clean and press and snatch are the two standardized Olympic events in this competition.

Power Lifting is a competitive sport where the goal is to lift the greatest amount of weight from three exercises (bench press, squat, and dead lift).

Weight Training is an exercise program where free or stationary weights are used for the purposes of increasing strength, endurance, flexibility, skill, and power.

Body Building is an exercise program utilizing free or stationary weights to change body shape and form.

WHY DO PEOPLE LIFT?

The reasons people lift weights are as varied and numerous as the people who lift. The weight room may be the most democratic of settings in all of sports and society. People of both sexes, and all ethnic, socioeconomic, and age groups lift weights. The reasons may be to improve sport performance, improve physical appearance, improve fitness level, enjoyment of the physical activity, or a combination of the preceding.

BENEFITS OF STRENGTH TRAINING

The main attributes developed by strength training are muscular strength and endurance, power, flexibility, and body composition. Certain weight training programs can also lead to development in cardiorespiratory endurance. These basic elements of fitness are discussed in detail in chapter 3.

Strength is essential to a variety of everyday physical activities. Even though strength is a relative factor related to the demands of the activity, all individuals need a minimum level of strength. Those with low levels of strength run a greater risk of injury in lifting or while engaging in other physical activity. Performance in recreational sports and athletics is enhanced by high levels of strength. Strong abdominal muscles provide important protection against lower back problems. Strength training is also an essential part of physical rehabilitation. Common sports injuries such as tennis elbow, rotator cuff, ligament and tendon strains respond well to muscle strength programs. Better posture accompanied by more aesthetic appearance are also benefits from strength training.

BODY BUILDING

Many individuals lift weights to improve body shape and form and have little interest in athletic performance. Muscle size and definition take priority over strength and endurance gains. Body building refers to the body's morphology or form and structure that depend mainly on inherited or genetic factors. While your body type or build can be altered only slightly, substantial changes can take place in body composition by decreasing body fat and adding muscle mass. When you exercise you burn more calories than when you are sedentary; therefore you start to lose weight, provided your food intake remains the same. A strength and endurance program results in an increase of muscle tissue with a decrease in stored fat. Your body dimensions will change, resulting in a slimmer waist, trimmer hips and thighs, and improved overall appearance.

Table 1.1 lists in more detail the benefits that you may experience as a result of weight training.

ADAPTATION

The human body has an amazing capacity to adjust to and benefit from the many physical demands placed upon it. For example, the body is capable of adapting to many kinds of stress and even increasing its efficiency as a result of stressful stimuli. In the case of fitness training, research indicates that repeated physical stress (intensive training) will lead to increases in our functional capacity (strength and endurance). The main purpose in strength training therefore is to stress the body through a variety of exercises so that beneficial adaptations will occur. Strength training is only beneficial as long as it causes the body to adapt to the physical efforts. If the stress is limited, adaptation will not occur. If there is too much stress, then injury and deterioration will result. An important point to remember is that your physical fitness is largely a reflection of the level of your training. When you work hard, your fitness will be high. However, when you interrupt the intensity of the training, your fitness will decline. Further, individuals with low levels of strength and endurance can look forward to substantial gains in muscular strength and endurance after only a few months of rigorous exercise.

The unique thing about your strength training program is that you are completely in charge. You make all the decisions, set your own goals, and decide when and how to exercise. Your goals in strength training are very clear and measurable, with few ambiguities confronting you. Further, you are in a no-lose situation; failure is impossible. There are no records to break, no complex skills to learn; success is there for the asking. There is an immediate payoff; you will be visibly improved by your physical activity. Improved muscle efficiency will produce feelings of increased energy, health, and overall well-being. The benefits of training will be especially noticeable if you are in a poor level of physical condition when you begin your program.

Table 1.1

Benefits of Weight Training

Increase in:

Muscle strength

Muscle endurance

Strength of bones and ligaments

Thickness of cartilage

Capillary density in the muscle

Muscle mass (hypertrophy)

Longer duration of effort before exhaustion—stamina

Increased flexibility

Speed and power

Blood volume and hemoglobin

Muscle enzyme levels

Skill

Maximal work capacity

Equalization of muscle development

Decrease in:

Body fat

Stress and tension

Resting heart rate

Additional benefits may:

Help prevent injuries

Help rehabilitate injuries

Improve function of cardiorespiratory system

Alter metabolism to improve caloric utilization

Facilitate quicker recovery from workouts or competitions

Increase self-image and confidence

Improve appearance

Increase feeling of well-being

Naturally induce fatigue and relaxation

AGE AND EXERCISE

Exercise for older persons is a comparatively recent phenomenon brought about by a change in social mores and a new perception of the role of exercise in life. Exercise programs for older persons should consist of flexibility exercises, use of light weights, calisthenics, and continuous fast walking or jogging. Sudden rigorous bursts of exhaustive exercise such as sprinting or lifting very heavy weights should be avoided. Older people should concentrate mainly on endurance activities that are moderate and rhythmic in nature such as jogging, walking, swimming, bicycling, and light weight lifting.

Maximum strength of men and women is generally achieved between the ages of twenty and thirty-five, and significantly high strength levels can be maintained well into advanced age. Normally a progressive decline of muscle strength takes place with age due to a reduced muscle mass brought about primarily by inactivity. Physical training, however, can significantly modify the strength decrement with aging. Older persons can expect improvements when they begin to train in later life no less than younger counterparts.

Research is still limited regarding strength training in the aged. However, research is beginning to indicate that there are advantages to such programs. Between the ages of thirty and seventy muscle mass decreases by an average of thirty percent. Strength undergoes similar decreases. Fast-twitch muscle fibers show the greatest fiber atrophy in the aged. The losses of muscle mass and strength may be retarded and reversed by a strength training program (Frontera et al. 1988; Fiatarone et al. 1990).

Bone mass also decreases with age. Bone mass and density is regulated by loading. Loading conditions can lead to hypertrophic response in bone resorption. Strength training also enhances and preserves the durability, solidity, and wear resistance of joint tissue (Carter, Fyhrie, and Whalen 1987).

Finally, if you follow the individualized exercises and guidelines presented in this book, you will be following procedures based upon sound scientific principles, which will benefit your health, and also be a source of continued satisfaction and enjoyment to you.

Glossary

Body Building   Exercise program that utilizes free and stationary weights to change body shape and form.

Conditioning   The development of high levels of muscular strength and endurance and high levels of cardiorespiratory endurance.

Muscle Endurance   The ability of a muscle group to maintain a continuous contraction or repetition over a period of time.

Muscle Power   The product of strength and speed.

Muscle Strength   The amount of force that can be exerted by a muscle group for one movement or repetition.

Power Lifting   A competitive event where the goal is to lift the greatest amount of weight for three different exercises (bench press, dead lift, and squat). Explosive power is important in this event.

Weight Lifting   A competitive event where the goal is to lift the greatest amount of weight for two exercises (clean/press and snatch). Skill, speed, and strength are important.

Weight Training   Exercise program using free or stationary weights for the purpose of increasing strength, endurance, power, skill, and flexibility.

References

Carter, D.R., D.P. Fyhrie, and R.T. Whalen. 1987. Trabecular bone density and loading history. Regulation of connective tissue biology by mechanical injury. *Journal of Biomechanics* 20:785–94.

Fiatarone, M.A., E.C. Marks, N.D. Ryan, C.N. Meridith, L.A. Lipsits, and W.J. Ebans. 1990. High intensity strength training in nonagenarians, effects on skeletal muscle. *Journal of the American Medical Association* 263:3029–34.

Frontera, W.R., C.N. Meridith, K.P. O'Reilly, H.G. Knutgen, and W.J. Ebans. 1988. Strength conditioning in older men, skeletal muscle hypertrophy and improved function. *Journal of Applied Physiology* 64:1038–44.

chapter 2

elements of fitness

Objectives

After studying this chapter you should be able to:

1. Describe the importance of strength training.

2. Describe the basic elements of physical fitness.

3. Define muscle strength.

4. Define muscle endurance.

5. Define cardiorespiratory endurance.

6. Define flexibility.

7. Define body composition.

Our misconceptions about fitness are legend. Many people still find it surprising that professional athletes such as baseball players or golfers may have poor cardiorespiratory fitness. Others feel that vibrating and whirlpooling their muscles in a health club will insure fitness, or that by taking a short walk once a week, fitness will automatically be conferred upon them. Misconceptions stem partly from two different concepts of fitness: performance-related fitness and health-related fitness. Performance-related fitness refers to many of the tests you may have taken that measure your level of strength, skill, power, endurance, and agility in specific sports. These performance-related tests measure only limited aspects of fitness. Health-related fitness concerns those aspects of our physiological and psychological functioning that afford us some protection against coronary heart disease, problems associated with being overweight, various muscular and skeletal disorders, and the physiological complications of our response to stress. The President's Council on Physical Fitness and Sports defines health-related fitness as the ability to carry out daily tasks with vigor, without undue fatigue, and with ample energy to enjoy leisure-time pursuits and to meet unforeseen injuries. This definition means fitness is a relative term relating to your everyday activities. Some of us need higher levels of fitness than others (physical laborer or competitive athlete). However, all individuals must meet a minimum level of fitness to lead a healthy and productive life.

There are five major elements to physical fitness, and the training program you choose should be geared toward the development of these elements. They are muscular strength, muscular endurance, cardiorespiratory endurance, flexibility, and body composition.

STRENGTH (SKELETAL-MUSCULAR STRENGTH)

Strength is the ability of a muscle to produce a maximum amount of force. It is measured by the ability to perform one repetition of an exercise at maximum resistance (1 RM). An example of maximum strength would be the greatest amount of weight one can lift in the bench press exercise.

Strength is of major significance in many sports and sport skills. Strength is a significant factor in one's ability to put the shot, throw the javelin, have a high velocity tennis serve, throw a fastball in baseball and softball, and many other sport skills. Strength is also important in sport skills that require a large amount of force to be applied to an opponent, such as wrestling and football.

ENDURANCE (SKELETAL-MUSCULAR ENDURANCE)

Endurance is the ability of a muscle to produce force continually over a period of time. It is measured by the number of repetitions of the movement or skill. If a person can perform thirty-five push-ups, then push-ups are for him or her an endurance skill. If, however, a person can do only one push-up, then for him or her the push-up is a strength skill. The key here is that endurance is the ability to apply force repeatedly or for a prolonged amount of time. Examples of sports requiring endurance are rowing, wrestling, hurdling, sprinting, sprint swimming, and sprint bicycling.

An athlete can continue to produce muscular force for only a short period of time before the energy stored in the muscle is depleted. In movements that require maximum force (strength), this occurs very quickly (one or two repetitions). If less force is required (less than maximal), then the movement can continue for a longer period (endurance).

If the amount of force required of a particular muscle or muscle group is low and the movement is cyclic, allowing a brief rest period (during which another muscle group is producing the movement), then the blood stream can bring nutrients to the muscle cells, and the movement can be prolonged for long periods. Examples of such movement are distance running, swimming, and bicycling. The ability to supply the necessary nutrients to the muscle cells in this fashion is a function of cardiorespiratory endurance.

CARDIORESPIRATORY ENDURANCE

Cardiorespiratory endurance refers to the ability of the respiratory system (lungs and associated blood vessels) and the circulatory system (heart, arteries, capillaries, and veins) to supply oxygen and nutrients to the muscle cells so that muscular activity can be continued for prolonged periods of time.

Endurance events such as distance running, cross-country skiing, bicycling, swimming, crew, and triathlons are excellent activities for improving cardiorespiratory endurance.

The importance of cardiorespiratory endurance, aside from its role in sport success, is that it can significantly improve your cardiac risk profile.

Aerobic exercises such as running and bicycling are recognized by sport medicine specialists as important in the prevention of heart disease. Heart disease is the number one cause of death in this country, and we should all take steps to improve our risk profile. You should strongly consider including some type of cardiorespiratory endurance exercise in your program. See chapter 12 for more details.

While some sport skills rely more heavily on one aspect of fitness, most athletes need some measure of each of the three components of fitness mentioned (strength, endurance, and cardiorespiratory endurance) as well as flexibility.

FLEXIBILITY

Along with strength and endurance, flexibility is an important component of muscular performance. There are two kinds of flexibility, static and dynamic. Dynamic flexibility is defined as the opposition or resistance of a joint to motion. In other words, it is concerned with the forces that oppose movement over any range rather than the range

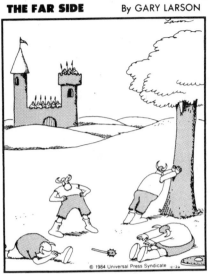

THE FAR SIDE   By GARY LARSON

© 1984 Universal Press Syndicate

The Vikings, of course, knew the importance of stretching before an attack.

itself. This type of flexibility is difficult to measure and has received little attention in exercise programs and competitive sports.

Static flexibility is defined as the range of motion that can occur at a joint. As a general rule you need enough flexibility to be able to go through the range of motion required for your sport or exercise without any restriction in the movement.

Stretching exercises can increase the range of motion of the joint. Weight lifting, if performed through the full range of motion, can also enhance flexibility. Flexibility exercises are often performed as part of a general warm-up prior to weight lifting. A general warm-up that includes flexibility exercises is recommended, particularly if you are stiff or sore from a previous workout or if the temperature is cold. A stretching program for weight lifting is included in chapter 13.

BODY COMPOSITION

Body composition refers to the proportion of body fat and lean body tissue to total body weight. The relative balance of these components is a better gauge of your fitness level than ordinary body weight. A recommended proportion of body fat for a man in his early twenties is approximately twelve to seventeen percent. For a woman in the same age group, about nineteen to twenty-four percent is recommended. Obesity is one of the most serious health problems confronting Americans today. Approximately thirty percent of all men and forty percent of all women weigh fifteen to twenty percent more than they should. Not only will obesity have a negative effect on physical performance, it also has important health ramifications. Being overweight is one of the major risk factors in heart disease. In addition, diabetes and high blood pressure generally accompany obesity. Physical exercise may reduce obesity and directly affect these two common problems. Obesity is also associated with gallbladder dysfunction, joint disease, and complications during surgery.

MUSCLE POWER

Power, which was discussed in chapter 1, is the ability of the muscles to produce high levels of force in a short time (explosive strength). Power can be increased by strength training and is basic to a number of daily activities and competitive sports. There is also a need for coordination and agility, especially if the need for the execution of power is in a particular sports skill such as rebounding in basketball or a lateral movement by a football lineman.

At this point you should think about the requirements of your sport or specific needs and also your strengths and weaknesses in that sport. Most people tend to work on their strengths, as this is easier and more self-satisfying. Working harder on your weaknesses, however, usually produces greater overall improvements.

Chapter 6 contains information to help you determine in which areas you are strong and in which areas of fitness you may require more attention.

Glossary

Aerobic (with Oxygen)   Refers to an activity in which demands of the muscles for oxygen are met by the circulation of oxygen in the blood.

Anaerobic   The process of energy production in which the oxygen supply cannot keep pace with tissue demands.

Body Composition   The proportion of body fat to lean body tissue.

Cardiorespiratory Endurance   The ability of the heart to deliver oxygen and nutrients to vital organs of the body.

Flexibility   The extent and range of motion around a joint.

Muscle Endurance   The ability of a muscle to produce force continually over a period of time.

Muscle Power   The ability of the muscle to produce high levels of force in a short time (strength and speed).

Strength   The ability of a muscle to produce a maximum amount of force.

1. Distinguish between concepts of muscle strength and muscle endurance. How can each be best achieved and for what purposes?

chapter 3

fundamentals of weight t...

Objectives

After studying this chapter you should be able to:

1. Describe the training goals in strength training.
2. Describe and define the basic principles in a strength training program.
3. Describe the sports training continuum.
4. Describe the process of selecting intensity of training.
5. Define progressive resistance.
6. Define specificity.

7. Define ... of foce.
8. Desc... ...ety procedures.
9. Defi... ...eating.
10. De... ...overload.
11. D... ...e repetitions.
12. ...fine duration.
13. Define frequency.
14. Define intensity.

The muscle system is the foundation of all physical exercise. No matter what activity you participate in, your muscle strength and endurance will significantly affect your exercise limits. It is also important to remember that your muscles are not independent from the rest of the body systems, and conditioning is not limited to the muscles. Your muscles' ability to do work is dependent upon the efficiency of the heart, blood vessels, and lungs in providing energy and waste product elimination. Muscles, the heart, blood vessels, and the lungs are simultaneously conditioned because of their interdependence.

More specifically, weight training goals may be directed toward increases in strength and power, in muscular endurance, or in a combination of strength and endurance. Strength and power training are important for power lifters, weight lifters, football linemen, and weight throwers in field events. Muscular endurance training is vital in order to increase the aerobic capacity of the muscles, which is required for activities such as cycling, swimming, and rowing. Finally, general conditioning exercises that aim to increase both muscle strength and endurance are vital for success in a number of sports activities. In addition, general conditioning prepares the muscle system to meet the everyday demands of individuals who are not involved in competitive sports. A large number of individuals also participate in weight training programs simply to increase the size and strength of their muscles for personal and aesthetic reasons. Regardless of your goals, a weight training program should incorporate the basic principles outlined in this chapter in order to derive the maximum strength and endurance gains in an efficient and safe manner.

Certain physiological principles need to be understood in order to develop a program that will turn your efforts into maximum gains.

Training is stress, and what we try to do while training is to apply stress in the correct amount with the correct frequency to achieve the maximum result. If we apply too much stress or apply the stress too frequently, with insufficient rest, then improvement will not be maximized. Improvement may even be hampered, and detraining (loss of gains) and injury can occur.

... d by the nervous system, a muscle fiber contracts ... stimulate. When stimu... at all. This means that an individual fiber, once ... produce by not con... all its force. We graduate the amount of force we ... nervous system. ... number of fibers we innervate or stimulate by the ... possible at one tim... strength, you try to innervate as many fibers as ... endurance, lighter lads... ifting heavy loads with few repetitions. To increase ... rest and recovery p... used and fibers alternate their contractions to allow a ... d, thus, a greater number of repetitions.

2. **Overload.** In order for... muscle to increase its capability, a greater load than normal must be applied... order for the adaptation to occur, a progressive increase in the amount o... k must be performed. Increases in strength require an increase in resistance. I... es in endurance require an increase in repetitions and/or resistance. ... adaption to this increased stress occurs, a greater stress must be imposed for ... her increases.

3. **Specificity of Training.** The gains... at occur from training will be specific to the type of stress imposed upon the s... tems. A lot of long-distance running will improve your cardiorespiratory endura... ce but will do little to improve skeletal-muscular strength. The opposite is also true, in that strength training yields little improvement in cardiorespiratory endurance.

4. **Use and Disuse.** As a muscle is trained, t increases in size and functional ability; it is said to hypertrophy. If training ceases, the muscle begins to detrain, decrease in size, and lose its newly gained capacity; in other words it will atrophy.

5. **Individuality.** Individuals often respond differently to the same exercise programs. Many factors affect training response, including heredity, nutrition, fitness level, motivation, health habits (e.g., rest and sleep), maturity, hormone and enzyme levels, and environmental influences.

SETTING UP A PROGRAM

After you have given some thought to your goals, the needs of your sport, and evaluated your physical strength and weaknesses, you can refer to figure 3.1 and tables 3.1 and 3.2. They outline the methods and goals of various weight training programs.

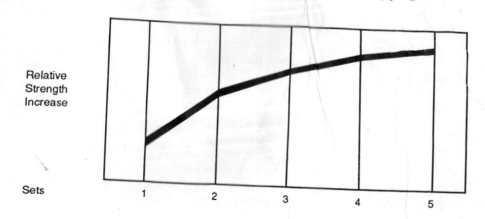

Figure 3.1
RELATIONSHIP BETWEEN THE NUMBER OF SETS AND INCREASES IN STRENGTH.

Reprinted from Getting Stronger *by Bill Pearl and Gary T. Moran. Copyright © 1986 Shelter Publications, Inc., Bolinas, CA. Reprinted by permission.*

chapter 3

fundamentals of weight training

Objectives
After studying this chapter you should be able to:

1. Describe the training goals in strength training.
2. Describe and define the basic principles in a strength training program.
3. Describe the sports training continuum.
4. Describe the process of selecting intensity of training.
5. Define progressive resistance.
6. Define specificity.
7. Define application of force.
8. Describe safety procedures.
9. Define cheating.
10. Define overload.
11. Define repetitions.
12. Define duration.
13. Define frequency.
14. Define intensity.

The muscle system is the foundation of all physical exercise. No matter what activity you participate in, your muscle strength and endurance will significantly affect your exercise limits. It is also important to remember that your muscles are not independent from the rest of the body systems, and conditioning is not limited to the muscles. Your muscles' ability to do work is dependent upon the efficiency of the heart, blood vessels, and lungs in providing energy and waste product elimination. Muscles, the heart, blood vessels, and the lungs are simultaneously conditioned because of their interdependence.

More specifically, weight training goals may be directed toward increases in strength and power, in muscular endurance, or in a combination of strength and endurance. Strength and power training are important for power lifters, weight lifters, football linemen, and weight throwers in field events. Muscular endurance training is vital in order to increase the aerobic capacity of the muscles, which is required for activities such as cycling, swimming, and rowing. Finally, general conditioning exercises that aim to increase both muscle strength and endurance are vital for success in a number of sports activities. In addition, general conditioning prepares the muscle system to meet the everyday demands of individuals who are not involved in competitive sports. A large number of individuals also participate in weight training programs simply to increase the size and strength of their muscles for personal and aesthetic reasons. Regardless of your goals, a weight training program should incorporate the basic principles outlined in this chapter in order to derive the maximum strength and endurance gains in an efficient and safe manner.

Certain physiological principles need to be understood in order to develop a program that will turn your efforts into maximum gains.

Training is stress, and what we try to do while training is to apply stress in the correct amount with the correct frequency to achieve the maximum result. If we apply too much stress or apply the stress too frequently, with insufficient rest, then improvement will not be maximized. Improvement may even be hampered, and detraining (loss of gains) and injury can occur.

PRINCIPLES

1. **All-or-None.** When stimulated by the nervous system, a muscle fiber contracts fully, or it does not contract at all. This means that an individual fiber, once stimulated, contracts with all its force. We graduate the amount of force we produce by regulating the number of fibers we innervate or stimulate by the nervous system. To increase strength, you try to innervate as many fibers as possible at one time, thus lifting heavy loads with few repetitions. To increase endurance, lighter loads are used and fibers alternate their contractions to allow a rest and recovery period and, thus, a greater number of repetitions.

2. **Overload.** In order for the muscle to increase its capability, a greater load than normal must be applied. In order for the adaptation to occur, a progressive increase in the amount of work must be performed. Increases in strength require an increase in resistance. Increases in endurance require an increase in repetitions and/or resistance. As an adaption to this increased stress occurs, a greater stress must be imposed for further increases.

3. **Specificity of Training.** The gains that occur from training will be specific to the type of stress imposed upon the systems. A lot of long-distance running will improve your cardiorespiratory endurance but will do little to improve skeletal-muscular strength. The opposite is also true, in that strength training yields little improvement in cardiorespiratory endurance.

4. **Use and Disuse.** As a muscle is trained, it increases in size and functional ability; it is said to hypertrophy. If training ceases, the muscle begins to detrain, decrease in size, and lose its newly gained capacity; in other words it will atrophy.

5. **Individuality.** Individuals often respond differently to the same exercise programs. Many factors affect training response, including heredity, nutrition, fitness level, motivation, health habits (e.g., rest and sleep), maturity, hormone and enzyme levels, and environmental influences.

SETTING UP A PROGRAM

After you have given some thought to your goals, the needs of your sport, and evaluated your physical strength and weaknesses, you can refer to figure 3.1 and tables 3.1 and 3.2. They outline the methods and goals of various weight training programs.

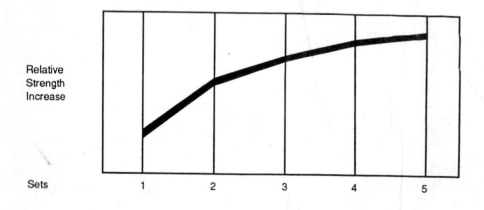

Relative Strength Increase

Sets   1   2   3   4   5

Figure 3.1
RELATIONSHIP BETWEEN THE NUMBER OF SETS AND INCREASES IN STRENGTH.

Reprinted from Getting Stronger *by Bill Pearl and Gary T. Moran. Copyright © 1986 Shelter Publications, Inc., Bolinas, CA. Reprinted by permission.*

Table 3.1

Sports Training Continuum		
	Strength training	**All around sports training**	**Muscular endurance training**
Goal	Strength & power	General conditioning (strength + endurance)	Muscular endurance (stamina)
Who trains this way	Power lifters Olympic lifters Football linemen Shot putters Others	Most athletes General population	Swimmers Rowers Cyclists Distance runners Cross-country skiers Others
Physiological changes	Increase in size of muscle fiber	Some increase in both size of muscle fiber and vascularization	Increase in vascularization, blood supply to muscle
Type of lifting	Low reps (2–4–6) Heavy weights	Medium reps (8–10–12) Medium weights	High reps (15–25) Light weights

Source: Reprinted from *Getting Stronger* by Bill Pearl and Gary Moran © 1986 Shelter Publications, Inc., Bolinas, California. Reprinted by permission.

Strength Training

The participants in this type of program are competitive weight lifters such as Olympic weight lifters, who perform the clean and press and snatch lifts, and power lifters, who specialize in three lifts: bench press, squat, and dead lift. This program is also used by power athletes such as football linemen, shot putters, and discus throwers.

These groups of athletes need a large amount of strength to be successful in competition. Their program is designed to increase strength. These athletes lift heavy weights for only a few repetitions, about two to six. When this type of training program is followed, the physiological changes that occur are an increase in the size of the individual muscle fiber and an increase in the ability of the nervous system to stimulate contraction of these fibers. These changes result in an increase in the force produced by the muscle.

Muscular Endurance Training

This program is used by endurance athletes to improve their stamina. The training program is designed to increase the size and number of blood vessels (vascularization) in the muscle and increase the efficiency of the heart and lungs. These changes are a function of increased muscular endurance and are achieved by doing many repetitions, about fifteen to twenty-five with light weights. This process pumps large amounts of blood into the muscle, which increases muscle size. The process is known as pumping. Pumping produces significant increases in muscular endurance but only minimal increase in strength.

Body Building

Many successful body builders started out as power lifters or Olympic lifters, acquired significant muscle fiber size, and then switched their program to a body building regime involving pumping action to achieve their massive muscular definition and development. Many body builders will use a strength (power lifting) program during portions of the year and then switch to the endurance program (body building) for competitive portion of the year. This regimen allows them to increase both fiber and vascularization.

Table 3.2

A Summary of the Methods of Weight Training for Various Objectives (Using Free Weights)				
Variable	Power	Strength	Local muscular endurance	Size
Sets	4–6	4–6	Maximum	4–6
Repetitions**	3–8	3–8	25–40	Varies*
Method	Explosive, using compensatory acceleration	Moderate cadence	Slow, continuous cadence	Varies*
Rest intervals	Short pause with relaxation between reps, and 2–6 minutes between sets	Short pause with relaxation between reps, and 2–6 minutes between sets	Allow heart rate to return to manageable level between sets	Varies*

*In size training, variation is the key; for maximal size, use all of the methods listed, interspersing them through each set or between sets. For power lifters, size resulting from increased contracting elements of a muscle cell (strength system using about 8 reps per set) is most appropriate.

**In deference to the principle of overload, you should always attempt to use the appropriate amount of resistance. The last repetition in each set should be a near-maximal effort. For strength and power training the resistance should exceed 80 percent of your maximum capacity, for muscular endurance above 40 percent, and for size it should vary.

Source: Fredrick Hatfield, *Power Lifting, A Scientific Approach*. Contemporary Books, 1985.

Sport Training

Sport training is the type of weight training that is performed by most competitive athletes. This program is recommended for those individuals interested in maintaining fitness for everyday activities and informal sport and recreation. Table 3.2 summarizes weight training methods with various objectives. (Refer to appendix A for more information on this topic.)

Most sports require a combination of strength, muscular endurance, and some measure of cardiorespiratory endurance. Most athletes benefit from a weight training program that yields gains in both strength and muscular endurance. This program is achieved by using a medium amount of resistance and performing a medium number of repetitions, about eight to twelve. The physiological changes that occur with this program are an increase in muscle fiber size and an increase in vascularization.

The sport training program is recommended as an initial or beginning program, even if one's goal is power lifting or body building. Also, if you have never lifted weights or are just returning to lifting, it is recommended that you follow a sport training program, as it will allow you to introduce your skeletal-muscular system and cardiorespiratory system to the rigors of resistance training without the levels of stress that the more specific programs (power lifting and endurance training) would place on you.

Power lifting places enormous stress upon tendons and ligaments as well as the muscle cells. These tissues need time to adjust to these high levels of stress, or injury can occur. Endurance training, because of its high repetitions, produces enormous quantities of biochemical fatigue products from cell metabolism. The buildup of these substances can cause significant muscle soreness, fatigue, and limited mobility. Because it takes time for vascularization to develop, you should work up to endurance training by first following a sport training program. Continue a sport training program for eight to ten weeks before shifting toward a strength or endurance program.

Before starting your exercise program you must be aware of three basic principles: intensity, duration, and frequency. Intensity refers to the degree of overload or stressfulness of the exercise, duration is the amount of time utilized for each exercise bout, and frequency is the number of exercises per week. Generally, the more intense, the longer, and more frequent the training program, the greater the benefits. Intensity and duration are interrelated, with the total amount of work accomplished being the important factor.

Selecting the Amount of Weight

2. Why is it advisable to begin with a sport training program regardless of whether or not one's eventual goal requires power lifting or endurance training?

Generally, to increase muscle strength, the intensity of effort should be near maximum with a low number of repetitions, and to gain muscle endurance, the intensity of effort should be lower with a high number of repetitions. The intensity level for strength gains is believed to be between one and six repetitions maximum. One repetition maximum (1 RM) is the maximum load that you can lift successfully one time through the full range of movement, two repetitions maximum (2 RM) is the amount you can lift successfully two times through the full range of movement, and so on.

Weight training research indicates that weight loads exceeding seventy-five percent of maximum are necessary for promoting strength gains, because the most important factor in strength development is intensity. Ten RM weight load usually corresponds to about seventy-five percent of that maximum.

An important factor in beginning your program is selection of the appropriate weight that should be lifted. The key is to select the amount of weight that allows you to perform the right number of repetitions for your program. For example, in the sport training program, we recommend that you perform three sets of the following repetitions (10-10-10).

Set 1—10 repetitions
Set 2—10 repetitions
Set 3—10 repetitions

You should choose a weight for set 1 that you can lift ten times (repetitions). You should work hard to perform the tenth repetition. If you could have done more repetitions, then the weight was too light. If you were able to do only six, eight, or nine repetitions, then the weight was too heavy.

The first few weight lifting sessions will be primarily testing sessions to determine the proper weight that you should lift. It is important that you keep accurate records (see record card, appendix E) and have someone spot you during this period.

After your first set of ten repetitions, you should rest from one to two minutes before your second set. You may find that on your second set you are able to perform twelve repetitions of the same weight you used for the first set. If this occurs, then you will need to add weight (five to ten lbs.) for the second set to bring your repetitions down to ten. The same may occur with your third set. This increase in strength often occurs and is a result of the influx of blood and increased nerve stimulation to the muscle, making it better able to respond to the demands you make upon it.

To restate our example then, your program might look like this:

Set 1	10 repetitions	X amount of weight
Set 2	10 repetitions	X plus 5 pounds
Set 3	10 repetitions	X plus 10 pounds

Again, please note that the key to the program is the number of repetitions. If, after ten weeks, you want to shade your sport training program towards *strength development,* then you might do 3 sets of 8 repetitions or a program as follows:

Set 1	10 repetitions	X amount of weight
Set 2	8 repetitions	X plus 10 pounds
Set 3	8 repetitions	X plus 15 pounds

If, after ten weeks of a sport conditioning program, you wanted to shade your program towards *endurance development,* you might choose the following type of program:

Set 1	10 repetitions	X amount of weight
Set 2	12 repetitions	X amount of weight
Set 3	12 repetitions	X plus 5 pounds

After you have followed the sport training program for eight to ten weeks, then your skeletal-muscular and cardiorespiratory systems will be in better condition to shift toward a strength or endurance program if you so desire.

Remember! The number of repetitions and the appropriate amount of weight determine whether you are performing a strength, general, or endurance program, not how hard you work. How hard you work will determine your level of success and the amount of gain you achieve. We assume you are willing to work hard, or you would not be reading this book.

Remember the continuum:

Strength Development	2–4–6 repetitions
Sport Training	8–10–12 repetitions
Endurance Development	15–25 repetitions

3. Discuss the differences and interrelatedness among the basic principles of intensity, duration, and frequency. In order to promote gains in strength, which factor is the most important?

How Often Should You Lift?

The general rule for weight lifting is to exercise the various muscle groups three times per week. Just as in a running or bicycling program, the best results are achieved when stress is applied in a hard day/easy day fashion. This approach allows for cellular changes to occur at an optimum rate and avoids overstressing or overtraining. In weight training we follow the hard/easy system by working hard one day and then following it with a day off. So a three-day-a-week program would follow a M–W–F or T–Th–Sat routine. The off-days allow the muscles time to recover from the stress that lifting imposes upon them.

Many experienced weight lifters lift more than three times per week (e.g., six days per week), but they will exercise a body part only three times per week. In this program the lifter would work his chest, back, and shoulders on M–W–F and his legs and arms on T–Th–Sat. This way each body part is exercised three times per week with a day off in between. This program is called a split-routine and is performed primarily by advanced lifters who perform multiple sets of multiple exercises for a specific body part. Examples of these exercises include regular bench press, inclined bench press, and declined bench press for chest development.

In summary, you should work each body part three times per week. You can do so in a routine in which you do all of your desired exercises three times per week, or a split routine in which you perform a portion of your exercises three times per week and the remaining portion on the alternate days. For the beginning lifter, we recommend exercising three times per week, as it is mentally easier to gear yourself up to three workouts per week than six sessions per week.

How Many Sets?

Research in the area of weight training and strength development has found that three to five sets of an exercise produce the most gains. Figure 3.2 demonstrates the effect of various numbers of sets on strength development.

As seen in figure 3.1 you will experience gains with one set and even greater gains with two and three sets. After three sets there is a leveling off of the gains. Performing four or five sets of an exercise produces more gains than three sets, but the amount of this increase is less than occurs during the first three sets. In other words, you have to work harder for fewer results after three sets than you do for the first three sets. The law of diminishing returns prevails. Our recommendation is that you perform three sets of your major exercises. After you are conditioned to the exercises and want greater results, then you can go up to five sets. After five sets the curve flattens out, and little is gained for your efforts.

Overload

Muscle strength develops only when muscles are *overloaded*—forced to contract at maximum or near maximum tension. Muscle contractions at these tension levels

Figure 3.2
NUMBER OF REPETITIONS AT
VARIOUS INTENSITIES.

From Powerlifting: A Scientific Approach
*by Frederick C. Hatfield, Ph.D. Copyright
© 1985 Contemporary Books, Inc.
Reprinted by permission of Contemporary
Books, Inc.*

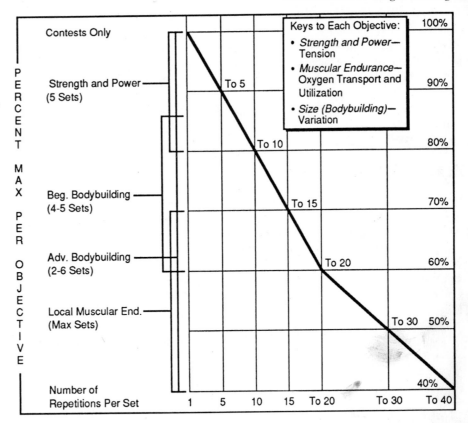

produce physiological changes in the muscles, resulting in strength gains. If muscles are not overloaded to this degree, they do not increase in strength or in size (hypertrophy). Muscles adapt only to the load they are subjected to. A maximum overload results in maximum strength gains, whereas a minimum overload produces only minimum strength gains.

Progressive Resistance Exercise

4. How can you determine whether you are performing a strength, general, or endurance program?

Credit for the development of the first progressive resistance exercise program goes to Milo of Greece, 300 B.C. Milo picked up a calf each day as it grew into a full grown bull. Milo progressively lifted a heavier weight each day to overload the muscles and stimulate the muscles to build greater strength. The resistance progressively increased as the calf grew each day and stimulated strength increase. Likewise, the intensity of the load you lift must be progressively increased to insure future strength gains. If the intensity of the training load is not increased, only existing strength levels are maintained. With progressive overload the muscle responds with an increase in size (hypertrophy) and strength. The same overload response can be used to increase muscular endurance by progressively increasing the number of repetitions performed or the amount of resistance used. If training stops, the lack of stimulus will result in a loss of size (atrophy) and strength.

Specificity

5. If you were to emulate Milo by lifting a heavier weight each day, could you continue to do so indefinitely? Explain your answer.

The demands of the exercise must be sufficient to force muscles to adapt, and subsequent muscle adaptations are specific to the type of training performance. This concept is known as *specificity*. For example, aerobic activity develops aerobic capacity, and anaerobic activity develops anaerobic capacity.

Recent research indicates that muscle adaptations are specific to the type of training performed because exercise not only affects muscles but also nerve control of muscles. The nerve pathways appear to become more efficient with continued exercise. The efficiency, however, is specific only to the particular exercise.

Research also indicates that the joint angle of exercise, the type of exercise (i.e., isotonic, isometric, or isokinetic), and the speed and range of movement all produce a variety of specific muscle adaptations.

Muscles will adapt specifically to the type of stress that is imposed on them. For example, strength training such as Milo's improves strength, while performing many repetitions increases muscular endurance.

It is important that you assess your strengths and weaknesses and the requirements of your sport so that you can train as specifically as possible to maximize your performance increases. (See chapter 6 and appendix A.)

Application of Force

It is also important to maintain a consistent application of force by raising and lowering the weight in a controlled manner. This type of movement subjects the muscles to the same level of stress during both the lifting and lowering phases. Generally the lift phase should take about one to two seconds and the lowering phase approximately two to three seconds. Fast movements require more strength at the beginning of the lift and less force during the later portion of the movement. High speeds of lifting and lowering are less productive in strength development, with the added possibility of causing injury to muscle tissue.

ORDER OF EXERCISES AND RECOVERY

Progressive training becomes less effective when muscles become fatigued, since the training stimulus cannot be maintained at maximum level. Also, overloading a fatigued muscle may lead to soreness and injury. Therefore, follow three simple rules:

1. Exercise large muscle groups before smaller ones. Movements become fatiguing when the small muscles involved in the movement are fatigued. For example, when working the upper body, exercise the chest and back muscles before performing exercises that work primarily the arms or forearm. If not, the fatigued arm muscle may be the limiting factor rather than the chest or back muscles that you are trying to exercise.
2. Arrange your strength exercises so that successive exercises only minimally affect the muscle groups that were just trained previously.
3. Allow forty-eight hours between strength exercises for physiological recovery.

6. Why is it necessary to train specifically in order to make gains in a given sport?

Combination of Exercises and Balance

To promote muscle balance, flexibility, and injury-free training, opposite muscle groups known as prime movers and antagonists should be exercised. For example, one should complement a quadriceps exercise (leg extension) with hamstring exercises (leg curl). There is a recommended procedure for combining exercises. You should exercise opposite muscle groups such as chest and back during the same workout. This approach ensures balance and harmony of muscle groups that work together in a movement.

A javelin thrower uses his chest and anterior (front) shoulder muscles to throw the javelin and also must use the upper back and posterior (back) shoulder muscles to slow the arm down after the javelin is released. If he develops the chest muscles alone, then he runs the risk of a strength imbalance and injury to back muscles.

The typical combinations of prime movers and antagonists are:

Chest	–Back
Shoulder	–Lats
Biceps	–Triceps
Quadriceps	–Hamstring
Abdominals	–Lower back

Warm-Ups

Warm-ups are necessary to prepare the joint for the activity. Many lifters prepare for the joint movement by performing stretching exercises to move the joint through the range of motion. Often lifters perform a light first set to accomplish this. If you are cold and sore from previous workouts or have been inactive for a while, you should pay particular attention to your warm-up and include jogging and stretching.

Flexibility and Range of Motion

If you exercise through the full range of motion of the joint, you will maintain and likely increase your flexibility. Champion weight lifters and body builders are among the most flexible athletes. The key is to lift through the entire range of motion of each joint. Flexibility exercises are included in chapter 10.

Breathing

It is very important that you breathe in a cyclic manner, both inhaling and exhaling with each repetition. Holding your breath throughout the lift can cause oxygen deprivation to the brain and can cause you to pass out. Obviously, this could be dangerous when lifting heavy weights over your head.

Holding your breath with a closed glottis during performance of resistance training is contraindicated. Blood pressure as high as 480/350 mmHg has been recorded during a double-leg press. Elevated blood pressure during lifting places an additional pressure on the heart and blood vessels. The simple principle is to exhale while lifting and inhale while lowering.

When performing a lift, inhale during the easiest part of the lift, *momentarily* hold your breath during the most difficult part, and then exhale when you can comfortably do so. When performing the bench press, for example, inhale as you lower the weight to your chest, momentarily hold your breath while you begin to press the weight upward, and then, during the effort phase of the pressing movement, exhale. As the weights you use become heavier, the momentary period of breath holding may become slightly longer. *You should never*, however, *hold your breath throughout the repetition cycle.* During heavy lifts you need that momentary pause in the breathing cycle (breath holding) to provide a stable support and anchor for the contracting muscles.

If while performing the bench press you exhaled during the beginning of the pressing movement (instead of holding your breath momentarily), the chest would compress during the exhalation at precisely the time you need a stable platform upon which the muscles can perform their contraction and movement.

Positioning

When performing lifts in a standing position (curls, overhead press etc.), your feet should be a little wider than shoulder-width apart, and you should be balanced fore and aft. Many lifters find that wearing shoes or boots with a heel can help offset the shifting of their center of gravity when they lift heavy weights (see figure 10.8). Lifters sometimes use a board under their heels when performing squats to assist in balance. Hands should be placed approximately shoulder-width apart for most lifts, a little wider for the bench press. Thumbs should be wrapped around the bar to insure a stable grip.

Back

In most lifts, such as the dead lift and bent rowing, the back should be kept straight and the lift performed with the legs or arms. This method will help protect the back muscles from strain and injury.

Head

Keep the head and neck straight during almost all lifts. Twisting of the head, neck, and trunk causes injury, as the muscles are less efficient when the spine is twisted.

Safety

Safety should concern every athlete in the weight room. To be injured because you or someone else failed to exercise caution and lift safely is truly disheartening. Rules to follow include:

1. Warm up properly.
2. Do not try heavy resistance until you are familiar with the technique you are using.
3. Do not use heavy weights without a spotter (someone to help if you need help).
4. Collars should be used to insure that the weights do not slide off and unbalance the bar.
5. Do not jerk or twist when you lift as these movements significantly increase stress and risk of injury.
6. Use care when performing the following exercises:

   a. Full squats—The structure of the knee is such that this exercise can cause ligament and tendon stress in some individuals. Half squats, to a ninety-degree angle between thigh and leg, are recommended.

   b. Back hyperextensions—Back hyperextensions are a good exercise for strengthening the lower back, however; if too much weight is used too soon, the back muscles can tighten and spasm. Start with light weights and add resistance very gradually.

   c. Straight-leg sit-ups—Straight-leg sit-ups should be avoided as they place significant stress on the lower back. Sit-ups should be done with the knees bent to approximately ninety degrees or more.

   d. Dead lift—The dead lift is a good exercise for the thighs and buttocks, but you should keep the back straight and lift with the legs. You should keep your head up and eyes on the ceiling; squeeze your buttocks and tighten your abdominals when performing this lift.

7. Too much velocity generated while lifting may prove to be dangerous. Excessive speeds at the end of motion of a joint may result in loss of control and tissue damage.

EQUIPMENT

Many lifters use various accessories to aid their performance and safe lifting. These include:

1. Weight lifting shoes or boots to aid stability.
2. Weight lifting belt to support the lower back.
3. Weight lifting gloves to insure a good grip and prevent blisters.
4. Weight lifting chalk used on hands to insure a good grip, especially when hands are wet.

Belts

Belts are effective in increasing intra-abdominal pressure, thus giving support to the spinal column while lifting. For resistance exercises not stressing the back, a belt is unnecessary. The belt should be worn for near maximal or maximal sets. During light sets

Table 3.3

General Principles

1. Warm up prior to lifting weights.
2. Include stretching exercises in your warm-up.
3. Stretching exercises should be done *slowly* through a *full* range of motion.
4. Do not try heavy resistances before you are familiar with the lifting technique you are using.
5. Include all the major muscle groups in your workout.
6. Insure that you involve opposing (prime mover/antagonist) muscle groups and aim for bilateral development.
7. For greater strength development, do fewer repetitions (eight or fewer); for a combined strength/muscular endurance response, work between eight and twelve reps.
8. Use a technique of lifting and a program workout that suits you personally—as long as it is wisely implemented. Vary the program in such a way so as to maintain interest in what you are doing.
9. Only by keeping accurate records (at least initially) can you effectively gauge your improvements and establish a routine.
10. Some caution might be taken while:
    a. Performing back hyperextension exercises with weights.
    b. Doing *full* squats.
11. Don't forget:
    a. Your weight training should be supplemented with an aerobic (cardiorespiratory endurance) activity, such as running, bicycling, or swimming.

it is not necessary to wear the belt. Beltless sets allow the abdominal muscles to receive a training stimulus, thus increasing their ability to protect the spinal cord. It is risky to suddenly perform lifting exercises without a belt if you are accustomed to wearing one while lifting.

Gloves

Weight training gloves are not required. However, they may be beneficial in preventing calluses and providing you with a firmer grip.

Shoes

An important factor in a weight training shoe is that it provides good lateral support. Running shoes with narrow heels and flexible shanks should not be used. Shoes that are designed for crosstraining or aerobic dance have a normal size heel and are more suitable for resistance training.

CHEATING

7. Describe the specific safety precautions that should be observed when performing each of the following exercises: Straight-leg sit-ups, full squats, dead lift, and back hyperextensions.

Cheating is the process of altering a lifting position to enable the lifter to lift more weight or to complete a repetition. An example is arching the back on the bench press. This arching changes the line of pull on the bone and transforms the flat bench press into a form of declined press. This procedure enables the lifter to handle more weight, as joint leverage is improved and the lower part of the pectoralis major is used more fully.

Another example is leaning back when doing the biceps curl to complete the exercise. Cheating is an advanced technique; novice lifters should use strict form on their lifts. Even advanced lifters should not cheat on all their sets but merely on the last few sets or last few repetitions of the last set.

Cheating is medically contraindicated. One should always proceed with caution because the increased joint motion can result in trauma to the tissue.

Advanced lifters use cheating to handle heavier weights than they can normally handle in the strict position. This step can result in their eventually being able to lift that weight with standard form. In short, there is a place for cheating, but it is for advanced lifters and should be used sparingly. Table 3.3 lists a summary of general strength training principles.

Glossary

Atrophy Decrease in size and functional ability of muscle.

Cheating The altering of the body's position to change leverage or use more muscle mass to complete a lift.

Duration The amount of time utilized for each exercise bout.

Frequency The number of exercises per week.

Hypertrophy Increase in size and functional capacity of muscle.

Intensity The degree of overload or stressfulness of the exercise.

Muscle Endurance The ability of a muscle group to maintain a continuous contraction or repetition over a period of time.

Muscle Strength The amount of force that can be exerted by a muscle group for one movement or repetition.

One Repetition Maximum (1 RM) The maximum amount of weight you can successfully lift one time through the full range of motion.

Overload Forcing a muscle to contract at maximum or near maximum tension.

Progressive Resistance The progressive increase in load intensity (either weight or repetitions or both).

Specificity The concept that exercises resemble the type of training performed.

chapter 4

general programs

Objectives

After studying this chapter you should be able to:

1. Describe a program to develop muscle endurance.

2. Describe a program to develop muscle strength.

3. Describe a program to develop aerobic capacity.

4. Describe a program for body building.

The following programs tables 4.1 through 4.4 have been selected for general conditioning for muscle strength, muscle endurance, and body building. You may make minor modifications to these programs depending upon how you respond to the exercise. Time is on your side, so don't overstress yourself for the first few weeks. Expect a little muscle stiffness and soreness the first few days. This is your body's way of telling you it has been a long time between workouts. This discomfort should go away in a short time. Tune into your body's signals while you exercise. You know more or less how you feel and how your body responds to exercise. You are the best judge as to what your body is capable of doing.

No single exercise can universally meet the needs of all individuals. However, no matter what exercise program you select, it should follow the sequence and fall within the time ranges shown in tables 4.1 through 4.4.

SPORT AND FITNESS CONDITIONING PROGRAMS

The goal of this program is to increase both strength and muscular endurance. This program is appropriate for most athletes and for those beginning a fitness program. The amount of resistance that is utilized will vary from individual to individual, but the principles remain the same. Perform this program three days per week.

You should consider supplementing your sport and fitness conditioning program with an aerobic conditioning program such as running, bicycling, or swimming. Perform the aerobic conditioning program three days per week, on days that alternate with those on which you do the sport and fitness conditioning program. (See chapter 12.)

After you have worked on the conditioning program for eight to ten weeks, you may choose to modify your program toward greater strength or muscular endurance development. The following two programs are designed towards those goals.

STRENGTH DEVELOPMENT PROGRAM

The goal of this program is maximum strength development. Perform it six days a week, following weight training program A three days a week, and weight training program B on three alternating days.

You should supplement your weight training program with a cardiorespiratory exercise program of three to five days per week in frequency. Your aerobic program should consist of ten to fifteen minutes of warm-up and flexibility exercises, twenty to forty minutes of aerobic exercise, and eight to ten minutes of cool down. You might

Table 4.1

Sport and Fitness Conditioning Program			
Weight training program (M–W–F)			
Exercise	Sets	Repetitions	Reference
1. Bench press	3	10/10/10	fig. 10.1
2. Seated rowing	3	10/10/10	fig. 10.6
3. Bent-knee sit-ups	1	25–75	fig. 10.17
4. Half squats	3	10/10/10	fig. 10.24
5. Triceps pull-down	3	10/10/10	fig. 10.15
6. Seated dumbbell curl	3	10/10/10	fig. 10.12

consider three days a week of cycling, swimming, or running as an adjunct to your weight training program. See chapter 12 for a circuit training aerobic program and appendix D for an aerobic running program.

MUSCULAR ENDURANCE DEVELOPMENT PROGRAM

Maximum endurance development (three–six days per week). This program can be done either as a regular routine, three days per week, or as a split routine, six days per week with upper body M–W–F and lower body T–Th–Sat. It is presented here as a split routine.

This program utilizes supersets, a system whereby you alternate exercises, a and b, followed by a rest. You repeat that sequence until the appropriate number of sets are accomplished.

You should supplement your weight training program with a cardiorespiratory endurance program three to seven days per week. You might consider three days a week of cycling and/or three days a week of running as a warm-up to the weight training program.

BODY BUILDING

Body builder programs are organized to increase muscle size, develop symmetry, and increase muscle definition. Body building programs contain more exercises than other resistance programs, as they focus on multiple exercises for various muscle groups. Body builders generally progress from exercising large muscles to exercising small muscle groups. The loads utilized by advanced body builders range from 1 to 40 RM. Beginning body builders use a range of 7 to 20 RM. It is important to insure a large volume of exercise during training. High-intensity volume is important in producing hypertrophy. Exercises usually consist of three to six sets. However, sometimes as many as fifteen sets of different exercises can be performed for specific muscle groups. Rest periods between sets are no more than two minutes and sometimes less than one minute.

Advanced body builders will focus on developing muscle mass through a strength training program (heavy weights, few repetitions) for part of the year or training cycle. This is followed by a medium weight, medium repetition program (8–12 rep) and finally a light weight, many repetition program (15–40 rep) for muscular hypertrophy and definition. This routine is the final stage before competition.

We caution the beginning body builder against incorporating the very heavy weight and/or very high repetition portion of this advanced program, as it takes years of training to develop the strength of muscle tissue, tendons, and ligaments to withstand such high stress levels and volume. The beginning body builder should stay in the 8–12 repetition range and cautiously work progressively toward the advanced program over time.

Remember, injuries slow or stop your progress; attempting to advance too rapidly ends up being counter-productive.

Table 4.2

Strength Development Program

Weight training program A (M–W–F)

Exercise	Sets	Repetitions	Reference
1. Bench press	5	10/8/6/4/2	fig. 10.1
2. Seated rowing	5	10/8/6/4/2	fig. 10.6
3. Military press	3–5	10/8/6/(4/2)	fig. 10.8
4. Lateral pull-down	3–5	10/8/6/(4/2)	fig. 10.7
5. Crunch sit-ups	3	15–25	fig. 10.18
6. Trips pull-overs	3–5	10/8/6(4/2)	fig. 10.13
7. Curls	3–5	10/8/6/(4/2)	fig. 10.11

Weight training program B (T–Th–Sat)

Exercise	Sets	Repetitions	Reference
1. Half squats	3–5	10/8/6/(4/2)	fig. 10.24
2. Sit-ups with weights	3	10–20	fig. 10.20b
3. Leg extension	3	10/8/6	fig. 10.30
4. Leg flexion	3	10/8/6	fig. 10.31
5. Back hyperextension	3	10–20	fig. 10.23
6. Toe raises	3	10/8/6	fig. 10.33

Table 4.3

Muscular Endurance Development Program

Weight training program A (M–W–F)

Exercise	Sets	Repetitions	Reference
1. a. Bench press	3–5	(18/16) –14–12–10	fig. 10.1
b. Bent rowing	3–5	(18/16) –14/12/10	fig. 10.5
2. a. Upright rowing or inclined bench press	3	14/12/10	fig. 10.9
b. Lateral pull-down	3	14/12/10	fig. 10.7
3. Alternating elbow to knee sit-ups	1	50–100	fig. 10.19
4. a. Seated triceps Dumbbell curl	3	14/12/10	fig. 10.14
b. Standing biceps Dumbbell curl	3	14/12/10	fig. 10.11

Weight training program B (T–Th–Sat)

Exercise	Sets	Repetitions	Reference
1. a. Leg press	3	15/12/10	fig. 10.25
b. Back hyperextension	3	15/15/15	fig. 10.23
2. a. Hip flexion	3	12/12/10	fig. 10.26
b. Hip extension	3	15/12/10	fig. 10.27
3. a. Hip abduction	3	15/12/10	fig. 10.29
b. Hip adduction	3	15/12/10	fig. 10.28
4. Bent-knee sit-ups	1	50–100	fig. 10.17
5. a. Leg extension	3	15/12/10	fig. 10.30
b. Leg flexion	3	15/12/10	fig. 10.31

Table 4.4

Beginning body building program

M/Th   Upper body—chest and back

Exercise	Sets	Repetitions	Reference
1. Bench press	3–5	8–12	fig. 10.1
2. Inclined dumbbell flies	3	8–12	fig. 10.2
3. Declined bench press	3	8–12	fig. 10.3
4. Bent rowing	3–5	8–12	fig. 10.5
5. Seated pulley rows	3–5	8–12	fig. 10.6
6. Pec deck	3–5	8–12	fig. 10.4
7. Abdominal exercises	1–3	25	fig. 10.17, 10.18

Body building program

Tue/Fri   Lower body

Exercise	Sets	Repetitions	Reference
1. Squat	3–5	8–12	fig. 10.24
2. Leg press	3–5	8–12	fig. 10.25
3. Leg extension	3	8–12	fig. 10.30
4. Leg flexion	3	8–12	fig. 10.31
5. Toe raise	3–5	8–12	fig. 10.32
6. Seated toe raises	3	15–25	fig. 10.33
7. Abdominal exercises	1–5	10–50	fig.10.17, 10.18

Body building program

Wed/Sat   Upper body—shoulders and arms

Exercise	Sets	Repetitions	Reference
1. Standing press	3–5	8–12	fig. 10.8
2. Upright rowing	3	8–12	fig. 10.9
3. Lateral pull-down	6–8	8–12	fig. 10.7
4. Abdominal exercises	1–5	10–50	fig. 10.17, 10.18
5. Tricep pull-over	3	8–12	fig. 10.13
6. Tricep pull-down	3	8–12	fig. 10.15
7. Seated tricep dumbbell curl	3	8–10	fig. 10.14
8. Standing barbell curl	3–5	8–12	fig. 10.11
9. Seated alternate dumbbell curls	3–5	8–12	fig. 10.12
10. Shoulder dips	3–5	8–15	fig. 10.10

chapter 5

motivation and mental conditioning

Objectives

After studying this chapter you should be able to:

1. Describe the importance of motivation in achieving muscle strength and endurance.

2. Describe guidelines for staying committed.

3. Describe the process of mental preparation in strength training.

4. Define attention, focus, and concentration.

Motivation is the energy and driving force behind what we do in life. Its absence accounts for poor performance, under-utilization of our abilities, and failure to achieve goals. Motivation lies at the heart of our decision to begin a task, to expend effort on the task, and to continue expending effort over a period of time. There is little use in maximized effort, however, unless we know where we are going. Motivation is, therefore, not only the energy that drives our behavior but plays a major role in establishing the goals toward which our energies are directed.

WHY WE DROP OUT

An important question that is often asked is, "Why is it so difficult for many capable individuals to unlearn poor health habits and form new ones?" Is there some undiscovered personality trait that allows some individuals to be able to complete a weight loss program, give up cigarette smoking, and run three miles three times a week? Evidence indicates that two important questions have to be answered before embarking on a program. First, what is the perceived chance of achieving the outcome, and, secondly, what is the value that is placed on the outcome once it has been achieved? Am I capable of achieving increases in strength, and if I do, of what benefit will that increased strength be to me? Regarding the first question, evidence indicates that some individuals are more confident that they will be able to achieve their goals. If you believe you are capable of attaining a goal, you are more likely to achieve it. When faced with obstacles, people who entertain serious doubts about their ability to achieve a goal generally reduce their driving efforts toward their goal or give up altogether. Factors such as past success and encouragement play a vital part of your perception of success. The more you believe your effort will help you attain your goal, the greater your chance for success. An important point to remember is that the low fit or sedentary individual can look forward to substantial gains in muscular strength and endurance in only a few months of rigorous exercise.

A second consideration is what value we place on the outcomes of our effort. Social science research shows that humans act to maximize gains and minimize losses according to their perceptions of what constitutes a gain or a loss. We will act to ensure benefits to our well-being. We have basic needs that determine why we strive, work, and persevere. These needs must be fulfilled for us to lead a balanced life and to achieve challenging but obtainable goals. We all enjoy the satisfaction of achievement whether it comes from making something with our hands, earning a promotion at work, or lifting an extra ten pounds. A sense of mastery, a completion of a difficult task, leads to a feeling of self-confidence and well-being. In addition, the physical and psychological benefits outlined in chapter 1 should be important to you.

On the other hand, be cautious about exercise dependence. For example, some people spend most of their waking hours in the weight room. They clock in more time in their workout shorts than street clothes. They become obsessed and set higher and higher standards, which require more and more of their time, and they lose sight of the important reasons for exercising. Do not strive for unrealistic goals. Place exercise in proper perspective to your personal goals in life. The purpose for most individuals is to improve themselves and to achieve a realistic self-concept.

A FEW TIPS FOR STAYING COMMITTED

1. Make a list of the physiological and psychological benefits you expect to achieve from your program.
2. Think about past successes in your life, how you achieved them, why they were important to you, and their significance in the long and short term.
3. Evaluate your chances of success by evaluating your present status, your capabilities, and your limitations. Don't underestimate your potential. Remember! No one fails when he or she exercises.
4. Think how a training program will benefit you. Are you convinced that the physical and psychological changes that result from exercise will be beneficial?
5. Set both short- and long-term goals. Be honest with yourself about what you can accomplish. Set realistic and achievable goals.
6. Plan a strategy by making a list of what you need to do. This book will help you in this area.
7. Find a support group; you might find it beneficial to exercise with one or more friends. A group can provide feedback and personal support.
8. Vary your exercises to avoid boredom. Introduce variation, be creative, select exercises that bring out new skills, and extend and challenge old ones. Music also helps.
9. Stay within your limits and don't be obsessive about exercising. Don't worry about missing a few exercise periods. Don't be awed by others with more strength. Individualize your program. Don't compete with others.
10. Record your progress. *Keep records but don't keep score.*
11. Be patient. Nothing worthwhile happens overnight. There will be slumps and bad days and temporary loss in skill. Don't expect instant success. Change will occur.

CHANGING BEHAVIOR

It is difficult to change behavior without addressing the underlying causes; otherwise the same problems come back along with a new set of problems. Also, many of our behaviors tend to be adaptive and not maladaptations to everyday events. That is, we tend to make adaptations that enable us to get through each day with a minimum amount of stress. Another difficulty is that when we attempt to change our behavior in a positive way, we tend to find ways to undermine it. Certain changes make us feel less free, and feeling free is often more important than concerns about our health. However, if we are presented with informed choices for behavioral change, reinforced by results that we can experience and measure, we tend to stay committed.

Setting Goals

It is important to establish goals so that your progress toward a healthier life can be observed and measured. In order to do this, it is vital to develop a greater awareness of yourself and your environment. Focus on your lifestyle and convince yourself that you are capable of self-assessment and of taking action in the process of moving toward your goals.

Many individuals attribute their failure to achieve goals to lack of ability. They tend not to try again or persist; they stop trying. Research tells us that the reasons for failure can directly affect the ability to carry on. The most common reasons are lack of effort, ability, task difficulty, and luck. It is important to remember that motivation is changeable and under your control.

Some important aspects of goal setting:

1. Select a goal you can definitely attain if you exert sufficient effort.
2. Remember your level of success in achieving your goal is directly linked to the amount of effort you exert. Your willingness to undergo some discomfort is vital to achieving your goals.
3. If successful or unsuccessful in realizing your goals, determine why.
4. When you have reached your goals, establish new ones.

Foremost in this procedure is the establishment of measurable short- and long-term goals. For example, short-term goals could be determining your target heart rate, degree of flexibility, range of motion, or the amount of resistance to use for weight training. Examples of long-term goals could be jogging a mile in ten minutes, reaching the recommended muscle strength for your age and sex, or reducing your body fat by 5 percent. It is also important to set new goals as the previous ones are reached.

Some Important Aspects of Goal Setting

1. Establish your own realistic goals.
2. Put them in writing.
3. Your goal must be attainable.
4. Your goal must be measurable.
5. Your goal should have target dates.
6. Your goal should allow for change.
7. Your goal should state the amount of effort as well as outcome.

WHY DO PEOPLE LIFT?

The reasons that people lift weights are as varied and numerous as the people who lift. The weight room may be the most democratic of settings in all of sports and society. People of both sexes and all ethnic, socioeconomic, and age groups lift weights. They may lift to improve sport performance, improve physical appearance, improve fitness level, enjoy a physical activity, or a combination of some or all of the above.

Regardless of the reason or reasons, almost everyone who lifts weights experiences an improved self-image. Strength truly builds confidence. An increase in self-confidence can go a long way in improving one's sport performance, physical appearance, and outlook on life.

MENTAL PREPARATION

8. Achievement of short-term goals provides motivation to further progress. Prepare a record form for yourself on which you can chart your performances.

Today's athlete can find no more fertile area in which to improve his or her performance than that of psychological preparation. The importance of this avenue for improving both training and contest performance has been known for years. The Soviet and East German national teams have had a sport psychologist assigned to each team for twenty-five years. In the United States many professional and university teams use sport psychologists to help improve individual and team performance. In addition, many individual athletes not associated with teams are using sport psychology techniques and exercises to improve their training and performance.

We will concentrate primarily on the psychological techniques that are most pertinent to improve weight training performance, but we urge you to look further into additional techniques and exercises that may be pertinent to your particular sport or activity. A recommended reading list is given at the end of this chapter.

In weight training the majority of our efforts go towards training. Thus, if we can use some psychological techniques successfully, we can improve our training efforts, and gains will be greater.

ATTENTION, FOCUS, AND CONCENTRATION

The terms attention, focus, or concentration refer to the ability to direct our thoughts and efforts to a specific task and ignore extraneous stimuli. In weight training, you must be able to focus your attention on the lift in order to achieve maximum performance. This process is enhanced by limiting external stimuli that divert your attention and by narrowing your attention to the lift.

VISUALIZATION AND IMAGERY

One technique that can be useful in focusing your attention is visualization. It is commonly used by many athletes today. The process involves rehearsing the lift in your mind and seeing (visualizing) yourself performing the lift. You imagine through mental rehearsal the process of lowering the weight, the feeling of its weight, the power with which you stop the weight and change its direction upward, and the force of exertion as you press it upward. In your mind's eye you watch yourself doing this as you feel the sensation of doing so. You are rehearsing a successful lift. This is a particularly good technique to use when you are trying for a maximum lift.

POSITIVE SELF-THOUGHTS

One of the obstacles to better performance for almost every athlete is the recurrent appearance of negative thoughts. Negative thoughts occur because of the influence of past experiences, listening to the negative thoughts of others, or listening to our own self-doubts. The results of these inputs are that we often focus on a negative outcome rather than a positive outcome.

We often fail to lift a certain weight because we have convinced ourselves that we cannot do so. The way to deal with negative thoughts or self-doubts is to immediately change those thoughts to positive ones so that you are rehearsing success rather than failure.

The following are examples of changing negative thoughts to positive ones.

Negative thoughts	Change to positive thoughts
I can't . . .	I can do it. I have done it many times before.
I won't be at my best because . . .	I have done everything I can do to prepare.
The heat is so bad I cannot do anything . . .	The heat creates a greater challenge.
I am really nervous and anxious . . .	The last time I felt this way, I performed my best.
I am afraid that I will make a fool of myself . . .	Unless I face the challenge and take the risk, I'll never know what I can accomplish.
I don't want to fail . . .	What is absolutely the worst thing that could happen to me? I could lose. If so, I will work harder to try to prevent that.
What is the worst thing that could happen?	I will be disappointed if things do not turn out as I want them to; however, I'll work harder to ensure success.
You stupid jerk . . .	Why don't you try to do _____ next time? It might be a better approach than the one you are using now.
I don't think I am prepared . . .	I have practiced and trained hard for this performance so I am prepared to do well.
I am tired, I can't go on . . .	It is almost over, I know I can finish. The difficult part has passed.
I am getting worse instead of better . . .	I need to set daily goals and evaluate my progress on a regular basis.
I have failed to get beyond this point every time I have faced it . . .	I can learn from my mistakes. This time I will do what I need to do to be successful.
I don't care whether I win or lose . . .	I have put too much time and effort into preparing for this event not to put forth everything I can to be successful.
I lost again. I'll never be a winner . . .	I can learn from losing. I need to talk with a coach to get some help regarding those things I need to improve.
I will never be as good as . . .	With more work, I can improve my skills and my performance.
It is not fair. I work just as _____ but I don't do as well . . .	I may have to work harder than some to accomplish the same level. I am willing to work as hard as I have to because I want to succeed.
I never seem to be able to do this . . .	This time I am going to think through and mentally prepare so that I can do it . . .

Adapted from *The Athletes Guide to Sports Psychology,* by Harris and Harris.

There are many other aspects to sport psychology; the preceding was a brief introduction to the area. If you would like more information, we suggest the following books:

1. *The Athletes Guide to Sports Psychology: Mental Skills for Physical People.* Harris and Harris. New York: Leisure Press, 1984.
2. *Sports Psyching, Playing Your Best Game All of the Time.* Tatko and Tosi. Los Angeles: J. P. Tharcher, 1976.
3. *Peak Performance, Mental Training Techniques of the World's Greatest Athletes.* Garfield and Bennett. Los Angeles: J. P. Tharcher, 1984.

The following is a list of guidelines that you should follow during your exercise program.

Begin gradually and progress slowly. Results will show up in about two or three months; don't be in a rush.

Always check your heart rate during and immediately after exercise. Your heart rate response will tell you if you are doing too much, too soon, or too little.

Apply the Progressive Overload Principle. Gradually overloading a body system will lead to an increase in its capacity.

Exercise a minimum of three to four times weekly for thirty minutes or more. Exercise duration below this will not substantially increase your capacity.

Alternate light and heavy training. This will allow adequate recovery between workouts and reduce the risk of injury.

Warm-up before each exercise session. Warm-up will increase the work capacity of your muscles and heart and reduce the risk of injury.

Cool down after each exercise session. This will allow you to maintain the blood flow from the exercised muscles to the heart and decrease recovery time.

Use the appropriate training program outlined in each chapter. The start of your exercise program should be based on the outcome of your fitness evaluation found in chapter 3.

Glossary

Attention/Focus/Concentration The ability to direct our thoughts and effort to a specific task and ignore extraneous stimuli.

Imagery The mental picture we focus upon during visualization, such as the successful completion of a lift. These images help us in the process of performing our intended tasks.

Motivation The basic reason why we strive, work, and persevere toward our goals.

Visualization The process of forming a mental picture of an act that we will perform. Visualization can also be described as the act of rehearsing the successful completion of an act that we wish to perform.

chapter 6

evaluation and self-assessment

Objectives

After studying this chapter you should be able to:

1. Describe the importance of fitness evaluation.
2. Define muscle strength and endurance.
3. Define cardiovascular endurance.
4. Define body density.
5. Define flexibility.
6. Explain tests for muscle strength and endurance.
7. Explain tests for cardiovascular endurance.
8. Explain tests for body density.
9. Explain tests for flexibility.

It is essential that you make an objective evaluation of your present muscle strength and endurance in order to determine the focus of your training program. Muscle endurance is to some degree dependent upon muscle strength. However, it is possible to have a high level of muscle strength and a low level of muscle endurance. Also, this evaluation will enable you to set reasonable strength training goals and prevent unnecessary stress on your body's systems.

Also included in a complete physical fitness evaluation are tests of cardiorespiratory endurance, body composition, and flexibility. Because of the many variables necessarily found in fitness tests, such as sex, age, height, flexibility, and motivation, these tests are not precise measures and are subject to error. They should be used only as general guidelines for outlining your fitness program and as general indicators of how you compare with others of your age and sex.

MUSCLE STRENGTH TEST

Muscle strength can be easily assessed by the one-repetition maximum test (1 RM), the maximum amount of weight you can successfully lift once. Four tests are utilized: bench press (figure 6.1a and b), leg press (figure 6.2a and b), biceps curl (figure 6.3a and b), and shoulder press (figure 6.4a and b). For each, determine the greatest weight that you can lift just once for that particular lift. Begin with a weight that you can lift comfortably. Then keep adding weight until you can lift the weight correctly just one time. If you can lift the weight more than once, more pounds should be added until the true 1 RM is reached.

For each muscle group, divide the total amount of weight lifted by your present body weight in pounds to determine the percentage of weight lifted. Now find your percentages in table 6.1. This table is based upon the percentage of your body weight you can lift for each of the exercises.

(A more comprehensive muscle strength list may be found in appendix B.)

MUSCULAR ENDURANCE

Table 6.2 can be used to assess your muscular endurance.

The norms are based on a college-age population. (See chapter 10 for proper exercise positions.)

9. Why should an individual who is interested in strength training be concerned about endurance?

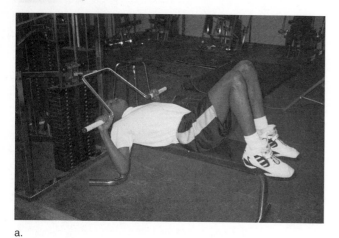
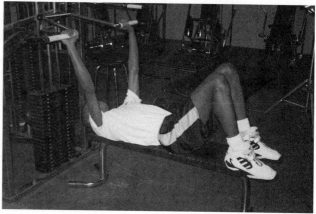

a.   b.

Figure 6.1 (*a*) BENCH PRESS (universal description).

From a supine position on the bench, grasp the bar with an overhand grip with the hands approximately shoulder-width apart. (*b*) Extend the elbows fully, but do not lock them. Progressively increase the weight until you can no longer make the lift.

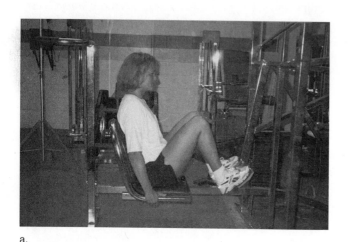
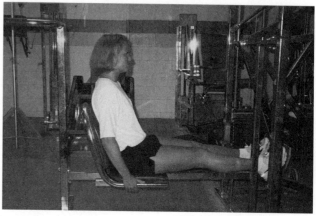

a.   b.

Figure 6.2 (a) LEG PRESS.

Place your feet on the pedals and grasp the handles on the seat. (*b*) Press your feet forward to elevate the weight and return. Inhale while lowering the weight and exhale while lifting it. Progressively increase the weight until you can no longer make the lift. Avoid hyperextending or locking knees.

PRECAUTION REGARDING THE ONE RM MAXIMUM STRENGTH TEST

Older individuals, those who have been sedentary for some time, and those with a low level of strength should not attempt the 1 RM test for maximum strength until approximately week eight of their training program. After eight weeks they will have developed sufficient skill, flexibility, and familiarization with lifting so that there is little chance of possible injury with the 1 RM test. The 10 RM level (see chapter 3) should be used in training up until the eighth week. Your 10 RM at a particular weight is equal to approximately seventy-five percent of your 1 RM. This can be used to estimate an individual's 1 RM in situations when a 1 RM attempt is inappropriate. Physically active college students may be given the 1 RM test during the second or third week. However, the test for muscular endurance can be safely administered during the first weeks of the training program.

Table 6.1

Muscle Strength Tests

Male	Percentage of weight lifted	Very poor	Poor	Average	Good	Very good	Excellent	Superior
				Fitness level				
Bench press	_____	50	75	100	110	120	140	150
Leg press	_____	160	180	200	210	220	230	240
Biceps curl	_____	30	40	50	55	60	70	80
Shoulder press	_____	40	50	67	70	80	110	120
Female	Percentage of weight lifted	Very poor	Poor	Average	Good	Very good	Excellent	Superior
				Fitness level				
Bench press	_____	40	60	70	75	80	90	100
Leg press	_____	100	120	140	145	150	175	190
Biceps curl	_____	15	20	35	40	45	55	60
Shoulder press	_____	20	30	47	55	60	60	80

Source: From *Health and Fitness through Physical Activity* by M. L. Pollock, J. H. Wilmore, and S. M. Fox. Copyright © 1978 by John Wiley and Sons. Reprinted with permission of the publisher.

Table 6.2

Dynamic Muscular Endurance Test Battery

	Percent of body weight lifted		
Exercise	Men	Women	Repetitions (max = 15)
Arm curl	0.33	0.25	_____
Bench press	0.66	0.50	_____
Lateral pull-down	0.66	0.50	_____
Triceps extension	0.33	0.33	_____
Leg extension	0.50	0.50	_____
Leg curl	0.33	0.33	_____
Bent-knee sit-up			_____
		Total repetitions (max = 105) =	_____

Total repetitions	Fitness category*
91–105	Excellent
77–90	Very good
63–76	Good
49–62	Fair
35–48	Poor
<35	Very poor

*Based on data for 250 college-age men and women.
Source: Heyward, V. *Design for Fitness*. Minneapolis: Burgess, 1984, p. 47. Used by permission.

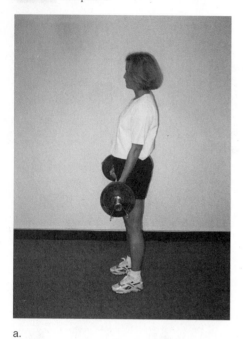
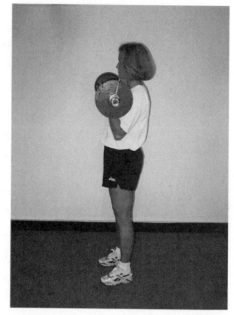

a.

b.

Figure 6.3 (*a*) BICEPS CURL.

Grasp the bar with your hands shoulder-width apart, using an underhand grip. Bring the bar to a position of rest against your thigh, with your elbows fully extended and your feet spread shoulder-width apart. (*b*) Using only your arms, raise the bar to your chest and then return to the starting position. Keep your back straight and always return to a position where your elbows are fully extended. Progressively increase the weight until you can no longer make the lift.

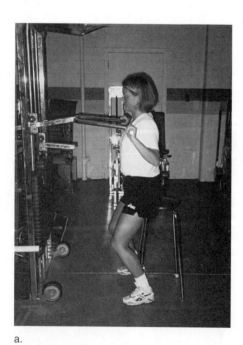
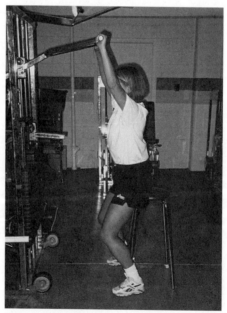

a.

b.

Figure 6.4 (*a*) SHOULDER PRESS (universal description).

Sit with your feet on the floor. Bend your knees and grasp the bar with an overhand grip, hands spread approximately shoulder-width apart. (*b*) With your elbows under the bar, assume a flat back, press the bar over your head as you exhale (do not forcefully lock elbows), and return to your starting position. Progressively increase the weight until you can no longer make the lift.

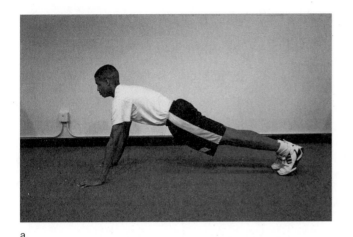 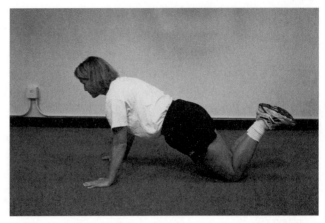

a.   b.

Figure 6.5 (*a*) and (*b*) PUSH-UPS.

Table 6.3

Push-Up Test

Standard push-up (weight on toes)

Age (years)	Superior	Excellent	Very good	Good	Average	Poor	Very poor
15–29	Above 51	51–54	45–50	35–44	25–34	20–25	15–19
30–39	Above 41	41–44	35–40	25–34	20–24	15–20	8–14
40–49	Above 36	35–39	30–35	20–29	14–19	12–14	5–11
50–59	Above 31	31–34	25–30	15–24	12–14	8–12	3–7
60–69	Above 26	26–29	20–25	10–19	8–9	5–7	0–4

Modified push-up (weight on hands and knees)

Age (years)	Superior	Excellent	Very good	Good	Average	Poor	Very poor
15–29	Above 48	46–48	34–45	17–33	10–16	6–9	0–5
30–39	Above 38	33–37	25–33	12–24	8–11	4–7	0–3
40–49	Above 33	29–32	20–28	8–19	6–7	3–5	0–2
50–59	Above 26	21–25	15–21	6–14	4–5	2–3	0–1
60–69	Above 20	15–19	5–15	3–4	2–3	1–2	0–

Source: From *Health and Fitness through Physical Activity* by M. L. Pollock, J. H. Wilmore, and S. M. Fox. Copyright © 1978 by John Wiley and Sons. Reprinted with permission of the publisher.

PUSH-UPS

Start in a standard "up" position for a full push-up, with your weight on your toes and hands. (If you have limited upper body strength, you can perform this test with your knees bent and your weight on your knees and hands.) Figure 6.5a and b illustrates both positions. Your partner should place his or her fist on the floor beneath your chest. Lower yourself until your chest touches your partner's fist. Keep your back straight while rising to an "up" position. Count the number of consecutively performed push-ups and then refer to table 6.3 to determine your fitness level.

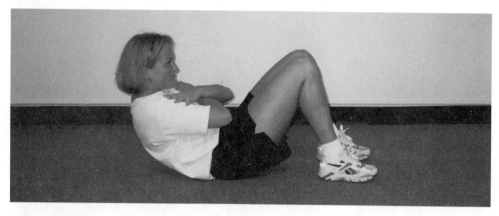

Figure 6.6 HEAD AND SHOULDER RAISE.

Table 6.4

| | | | Head-and-Shoulder Raise Score | | | | |
| | | | Fitness level | | | | |
Age (years)	Very poor	Poor	Average	Good	Very good	Excellent	Superior
Males							
17–29	0–17	17–35	36–41	42–47	48–50	51–55	55+
30–39*	0–13	13–26	27–32	33–38	39–43	44–48	48+
40–49	0–11	11–22	23–27	28–33	34–38	39–43	43+
50–59	0–8	8–16	17–21	22–28	29–33	34–38	38+
60–69	0–6	6–12	13–17	18–24	25–30	31–35	35+
Females							
17–29	0–14	14–28	29–32	33–35	36–42	43–47	47+
30–39*	0–11	11–22	23–28	29–34	35–40	41–45	45+
40–49	0–9	9–18	19–23	24–30	31–34	35–40	40+
50–59	0–6	6–12	13–17	18–24	25–30	31–35	35+
60–69	0–5	5–10	11–14	15–20	21–25	26–30	30+

Source: Reprinted by permission of the Cooper Institute for Aerobic Research, Dallas, Texas, 75265.
*The value of ages over thirty is estimated.

HEAD-AND-SHOULDER RAISE

Lie on your back with arms across your chest. Your knees should be bent at about ninety degrees with both feet flat and no more than eighteen inches in front of the buttocks (see figure 6.6). Don't forget to breathe, to assist in muscular contraction. Complete as many raises as possible in one minute. Warm up with a few raises before the test. Curl your neck and upper back until your trunk reaches a thirty to forty degree angle with the exercise surface, then return to the starting position.

Refer to table 6.4 to determine your fitness level.

MODIFIED SIT-AND-REACH TEST

The modified sit-and-reach test is an excellent measure of trunk **flexibility** (the extent and range of motion around the joint). (See figure 6.7.) Before attempting the test, warm up by jogging briefly.

Table 6.5

Modified Sit-and-Reach					
	Score at age				
	20–29	*30–39*	*40–49*	*50–59*	*60+*
Men					
High	≥19	≥18	≥17	≥16	≥15
Average	13–18	12–17	11–16	10–15	9–14
Below average	10–12	9–11	8–10	7–9	6–8
Low	<9	<8	<7	<6	<5
Women					
High	≥22	≥21	≥20	≥19	≥18
Average	16–21	15–20	14–19	13–18	12–17
Below average	13–15	12–14	11–13	10–12	9–11
Low	<12	<11	<10	<9	<8

Note. Reprinted by permission from *ACSM Resource Manual for Guidelines for Exercise Testing and Prescription* (p. 165) by S. Blair, P. Painter, R. R. Pate, L. K. Smith, and C. B. Taylor, 1988, Philadelphia: Lea and Febiger, which was adapted from *The Y's Way to Physical Fitness* (pp. 106–111) by L. A. Golding, C. R. Myers, and W. E. Sinning (Eds.), 1982, Rosemont, IL: YMCA of the USA.

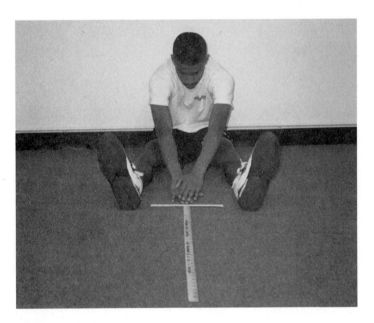

Figure 6.7 MODIFIED SIT-AND-REACH.

Method

1. Place a yardstick on the floor with the zero mark closest to you. Tape the yardstick in place at the fifteen inch mark. See figure 6.7.
2. Warm up properly using the "Easy Seven" in chapter 13.
3. Ask a partner to help you keep your legs straight during the sit-and-reach test. However, it is important that the partner not interfere with your movement.
4. Sit on the floor with the yardstick between your legs, your feet ten to twelve inches apart, and your heels even with the tape at the fifteen-inch mark.
5. With the index fingers of both your hands together, reach forward as far as possible, keeping your knees in contact with the floor.
6. Note the distance you are able to reach. Find your score in table 6.5.

DETERMINE YOUR CARDIORESPIRATORY ENDURANCE LEVEL

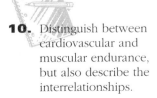

10. Distinguish between cardiovascular and muscular endurance, but also describe the interrelationships.

The chief means of evaluating cardiorespiratory efficiency is to determine the body's capacity to consume oxygen at a maximum rate. The assessment of oxygen uptake through laboratory testing is the most accurate method but requires a good deal of time and sophisticated equipment and is impractical for self-testing. The one and a half mile run test can be used to measure the amount of maximum oxygen uptake by determining the heart rate response to the exercise.

Table 6.6a

1.5 Mile Run Test	
Time in minutes and seconds	**Estimated max VO$_2$ in ml/kg/min**
7:30 or less	75
7:31–8:00	72
8:01–8:30	67
8:31–9:00	62
9:01–9:30	58
9:31–10:00	55
10:01–10:30	52
10:31–11:00	49
11:01–11:30	46
11:31–12:00	44
12:01–12:30	41
12:31–13:00	39
13:01–13:30	37
13:31–14:00	36
14:01–14:30	34
14:31–15:00	33
15:01–15:30	31
15:31–16:00	30
16:01–16:30	28
16:31–17:00	27
17:01–17:30	26
17:31–18:00	25

Adapted from K. H. Cooper, "A Means of Assessing Maximal Oxygen Intake," *Journal of the American Medical Association* 203 (1968):201.

Table 6.6b

1.5 Mile Run Test					
Age group (yrs)	**High**	**Good**	**Average**	**Fair**	**Poor**
10–19	Above 66	57–66	47–56	38–46	Below 38
20–29	" 62	53–62	43–52	33–42	" 33
30–39	" 58	49–58	39–48	30–38	" 30
40–49	" 54	45–54	36–44	26–35	" 26
50–59	" 50	42–50	34–41	24–33	" 24
60–69	" 46	39–46	31–38	22–30	" 22
70–79	" 42	36–42	28–35	20–27	" 20

[1]The average maximal O$_2$ uptake of females is 15 to 20 percent lower than that of males. To find the appropriate category for females, locate the score in the above table and shift one category to the left; e.g., the "Average" category for males is the "Good" category for females.

1.5 MILE RUN

The 1.5 mile test can be run on an oval track or on a straightaway. You should perform this test only if you have been training to run this distance and are in good physical condition. If you become overtired while running, slow down to a jog or walk. Do not unduly overstress yourself. Keep track of the amount of time it takes you to run 1.5 miles, and then find your estimated maximum oxygen uptake in table 6.6a and your fitness level in table 6.6b.

WALKING TEST

The walking test can be performed by low-fit individuals who cannot attempt the 1.5 test. To perform the test find a measured track or a flat course where you can measure a mile. Take time to warm up for several minutes, first by stretching thoroughly or walking. Your walking shoes should have a roomy toe box, flexible soles with good traction, and a stiff heel cup for stability. Running shoes have too much padding, which make your feet wobble.

Time yourself as you walk the mile as fast as you can without experiencing signs of exhaustion such as nausea or shortness of breath. When you finish, record your heart rate. (Take your pulse for fifteen seconds and multiply by four.) Cool down by walking slowly for a few minutes.

Table 6.7 will compare your current fitness level to "moderate" fitness. If you walk the mile in less time than the range shown for that heart rate, your fitness level is high. If it took you longer than that range, your fitness level is low. An older person needs a lower heart rate than a younger person in order to score as equally fit. This is because younger people have a higher maximum heart rate. They can end the test with a faster pulse rate and still have as much cardiac capacity and reserve as an older person who tests at a slower pulse.

If you fall within the moderate fitness range in table 6.7, then you can begin your walking-jogging program (appendix D) at starting level two to three (average). If your score is two or more minutes over the moderate fitness range for your age, your starting level should be one to two (poor-very poor). If you are two minutes under the moderate fitness range, your starting level is four to five (good-very good). If you are four minutes or more under, your starting level can be five to seven (excellent-superior).

TEST FOR BODY COMPOSITION

Body composition refers to the proportion of lean body tissue to total body weight. The recommended percentage of body fat for adult males is twelve to seventeen percent, for adult females nineteen to twenty-four percent.

The skinfold test for determination of body fat is based on the relationship of subcutaneous fat (fat just below the skin) to total lean body tissue. The method is subject to errors of as much as three to fifteen percent, plus or minus the actual body fat percentage.

To perform the test you need a pair of skinfold calipers. Hold the skinfold between the thumb and index finger. Release the tension on the calipers slowly so that they pinch the skinfold as close as possible to your fingers. Three measures are required for both male and female: the chest, thigh, and abdomen for the male, and the triceps, thigh, and iliac crest for the female. See figures 6.8 through 6.12.

After taking the three skinfold measurements appropriate to your sex, total the measurements on the nomogram in figure 6.13. Use the straight edge to connect the point on the left that corresponds to your age with the point on the far right that corresponds to the sum of your three skinfold measurements. Then read the percentage of body fat from the center male or female scale.

Table 6.7

Age	Heart rate	Time showing moderate fitness[1]	
		Men (175 lbs.)	Women (125 lbs.)
20–29	110	17:06–19:36	19:08–20:57
	120	16:36–19:10	18:38–20:27
	130	16:06–18:35	18:12–20:00
	140	15:36–18:06	17:42–19:30
	150	15:10–17:36	17:12–19:00
	160	14:42–17:09	16:42–18:30
	170	14:12–16:39	16:12–18:00
30–39	110	15:54–18:21	17:52–19:46
	120	15:24–17:52	17:24–19:18
	130	14:54–17:22	16:54–18:48
	140	14:30–16:54	16:24–18:18
	150	14:00–16:26	15:54–17:48
	160	13:30–15:58	15:24–17:18
	170	13:01–15:28	14:55–16:54
40–49	110	15:38–18:05	17:20–19:15
	120	15:09–17:36	16:50–18:45
	130	14:41–17:07	16:24–18:18
	140	14:12–16:38	15:54–17:48
	150	13:42–16:09	15:24–17:18
	160	13:15–15:42	14:54–16:48
	170	12:45–15:12	14:25–16:18
50–59	110	15:22–17:49	17:04–18:40
	120	14:53–17:20	16:36–18:12
	130	14:24–16:51	16:06–17:42
	140	13:51–16:22	15:36–17:18
	150	13:26–15:53	15:06–16:48
	160	12:59–15:26	14:36–16:18
	170	12:30–14:56	14:06–15:48
60+	110	15:33–17:55	16:36–18:00
	120	15:04–17:24	16:06–17:30
	130	14:36–16:57	15:37–17:01
	140	14:07–16:28	15:09–16:31
	150	13:39–15:59	14:39–16:02
	160	13:10–15:30	14:12–15:32

One-Mile Walking Test

[1]For every ten pounds over 175 pounds for men or over 125 pounds for women, time must be fifteen seconds faster. For every ten pounds under those weights, time can be fifteen seconds slower.

Source: Reprinted by permission of the Cooper Institute for Aerobic Research, Dallas, Texas, 75265.

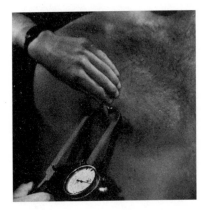

Figure 6.8 CHEST SKINFOLD MEASUREMENT.

Locate a point over the outside edge of the pectoralis major muscle just adjacent and medial to the armpit. The skinfold should run diagonally between the shoulder and the opposite hip.

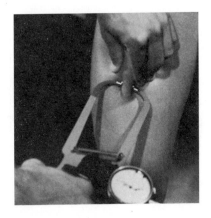

Figure 6.9 THIGH SKINFOLD MEASUREMENT.

Locate a vertical skinfold in the anterior midline of the thigh, halfway between the hip and the knee joint. Place your body weight on the opposite leg while taking the measurement.

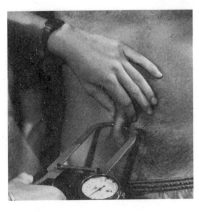

Figure 6.10 ABDOMEN SKINFOLD MEASUREMENT.

Locate a vertical skinfold adjacent to the umbilicus.

Figure 6.11 TRICEPS SKINFOLD MEASUREMENT.

Locate a vertical skinfold on the back of the arm halfway between the tip of the acromion process (bony projection on the tip of the shoulder) and the olecranon process (rear point of the elbow), with the arm hanging in a relaxed position.

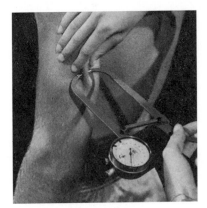

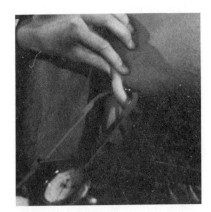

Figure 6.12 ILIAC CREST SKINFOLD MEASUREMENT.

Locate a vertical skinfold over the iliac crest (point of the hip) in the midaxillary line (middle of the armpit).

Table 6.8

Body Fat Score			
Male percentage of body fat	**Fitness level**	**Female percentage of body fat**	**Fitness level**
10	Very lean	13	Very lean
11–12		13–15	
12–14	Lean	17–18	Lean
14–15		18–22	
15–17	Acceptable	22–28	Acceptable
17–18	Fat	28–30	Fat
20+	Obese	30+	Obese

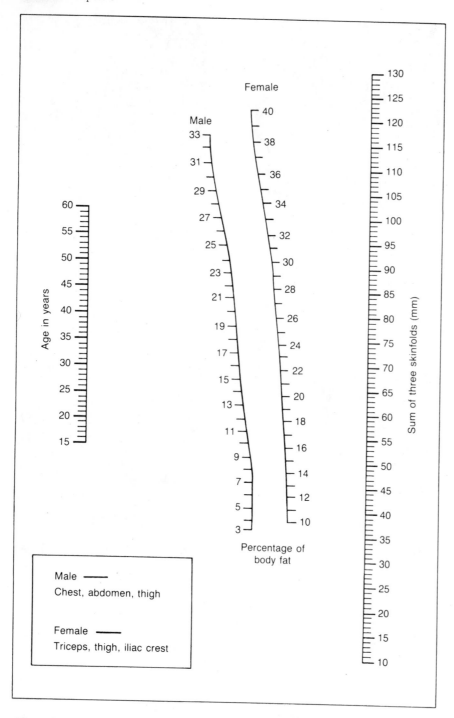

Figure 6.13

Nomogram for the determination of percentage of body fat for the sum of the chest, abdomen, and thigh skinfolds of males fifteen years of age and above, and for the sum of the triceps, thigh, and iliac crest skinfolds of females fifteen years of age and above. (See next page.)

Adapted from W. B. Baun, M. R. Baun, and P. B. Raven, "A Nomogram for the Estimate of Percent Body Fat from Generalized Equations," *Research Quarterly for Exercise and Sport* 52(1981): 380–84. Reprinted by permission of the American Alliance for Health, Physical Education, Recreation and Dance, 1900 Association Drive, Reston, Virginia 22091.

Figure 6.14

NOMOGRAM FOR
DETERMINING BMI.

B. T. Burton and W. R. Forster, Health
Implications of Obesity. An NIH
Consensus Development Conference,
Journal of the Dietetic Association, 85
(1985): pages 1117–21.

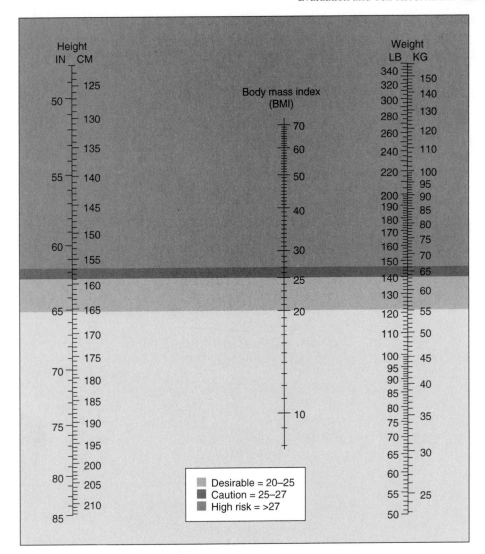

BODY MASS INDEX

If you don't have a skin caliper, **body mass index** offers an alternative way to define obesity. To calculate body mass index, divide your weight in kilograms by height in meters squared. The nomogram in figure 6.14 does this calculation for you. When the body mass index exceeds twenty-five, obesity-related health risks begin for men and women.

Mark your height and your weight on the corresponding scales, using a ruler or straight edge. Draw a line connecting those two points, then read your BMI from the middle scale.

Glossary

Body Composition   The proportion of body fat to lean body tissue.

Cardiorespiratory Efficiency   The ability of the heart to deliver oxygen to all of the organs of the body.

Flexibility   The extent and range of motion about a joint.

Muscle Endurance   The ability of a muscle to produce force continually over a period of time.

Skinfold Test   The method of estimating body fat by measuring subcutaneous fat with skinfold calipers.

chapter 7

muscles

Objectives

After studying this chapter you should be able to:

1. Describe the structure of a skeletal muscle.

2. Describe the physiology of a muscle contraction.

3. Define hypertrophy and atrophy.

4. Describe muscle soreness.

The basic function of skeletal muscles is to contract. This contraction enables human movement to occur. Over 600 skeletal muscles provide us with the capability to perform all manner of voluntary movement. Each voluntary muscle is a separate structure in its own right, containing connective tissue, nerves, and blood vessels. The muscles make up approximately forty-two percent of the body weight in men and thirty-six percent in women.

STRUCTURE OF SKELETAL MUSCLE

If you were to closely examine a skeletal muscle, you would find that each muscle has its own outer covering of connective tissue called epimysium. As seen in figure 7.1, the extension of the outer connective tissue at the end of the muscle forms the tendon, which connects and anchors the muscle to the bone. If the epimysium is peeled away from the body of the muscle, a number of bundles called fasciculi are revealed. Each bundle is surrounded by its own connective tissue structure called perimysium. Contained within this muscle bundle are the individual muscle fibers. Each fiber (some the size of a human hair) is surrounded by a covering of connective tissue called endomysium.

Each muscle fiber is composed of hundreds of cylindrical-shaped structures called myofibrils. A sheath or membrane covers each fiber, separating it from the surrounding fluid. The myofibrils contain the tiny protein filaments whose actions are responsible for the contraction of the myofibrils and, in turn, the muscle. The myofibrils are immersed in the fluid portion of the fiber called sarcoplasm. The sarcoplasm contains enzymes to power the mitochondria, which are the power packs of the cell. Myofibrils contain two kinds of protein filaments, thick ones composed of the protein myosin and thin ones composed of the protein actin. These proteins are geometrically aligned throughout the muscle.

As seen in figure 7.2, the smallest unit of the myofibril is the sarcomere, which is the distance between two Z-lines. When the muscle is stimulated by the nervous system, this small unit will contract. The A-band, the dark portion of the sarcomere, consists of both actin and myosin filaments with the actin filaments attached to the Z-lines. The tiny projections extending from the myosin filaments or the actin filaments are called the myosin cross bridges (fig. 7.3). These tiny cross bridges are instrumental in the shortening of the muscle. When the muscle contracts, the actin filament slides over the myosin filament toward the center of the sarcomere in a coupling process where the myosin cross bridges form a temporary bond with the actin filaments. This coupling process is dependent on the release of calcium ions stored in a membranous structure called the sarcoplasmic reticulum. Active sites on the actin filaments are covered by troponen and tropomyosin proteins. When the calcium ions are released, they bind with troponen and cause a change in tropomyosin so that it exposes active sites on the actin filament. When coupling takes place, the cross bridges swivel in a manner that causes the actin filaments to slide over the myosin filaments. This process activates the enzyme ATPase

Anatomy Chart

Muscles of the Body: Front. From Wayne L. Westcott, *Strength Fitness: Physiological Principles and Training Techniques.* Copyright © 1989 Wm. C. Brown Publishers, Dubuque, Iowa. All Rights Reserved. Reprinted by permission.

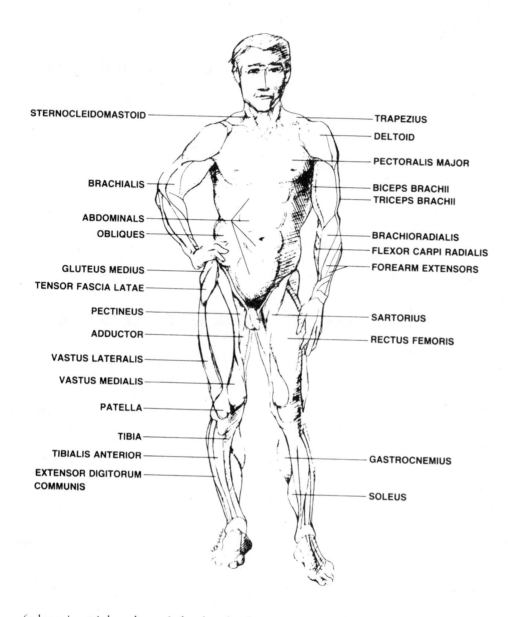

STERNOCLEIDOMASTOID

TRAPEZIUS

DELTOID

PECTORALIS MAJOR

BRACHIALIS

BICEPS BRACHII
TRICEPS BRACHII

ABDOMINALS
OBLIQUES

BRACHIORADIALIS
FLEXOR CARPI RADIALIS
FOREARM EXTENSORS

GLUTEUS MEDIUS
TENSOR FASCIA LATAE

PECTINEUS

SARTORIUS

ADDUCTOR

RECTUS FEMORIS

VASTUS LATERALIS

VASTUS MEDIALIS

PATELLA

TIBIA

TIBIALIS ANTERIOR

GASTROCNEMIUS

EXTENSOR DIGITORUM
COMMUNIS

SOLEUS

(adenosine triphosphatase) that breaks down ATP (adenosine triphosphate) stored on the cross bridges. ATP provides energy for the action between actin and myosin. For more shortening to occur, the cross bridges must break bonds already formed and bind to other active sites reloaded with ATP on the actin filament. This process is called recharging. When neural stimulation stops, calcium ions are pumped back into the sarcoplasmic reticulum, the cross bridges uncouple, and the muscle relaxes.

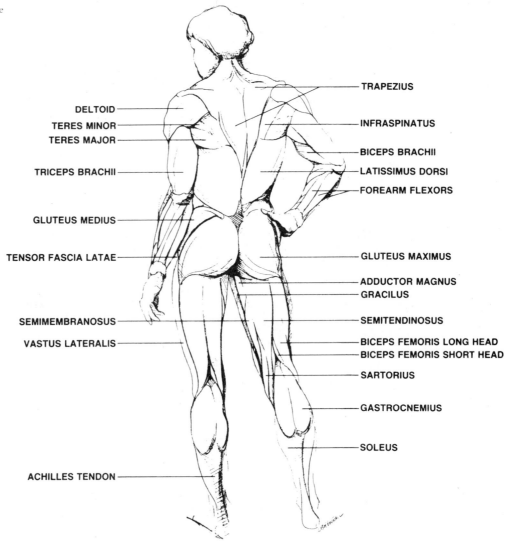

DELTOID
TERES MINOR
TERES MAJOR
TRICEPS BRACHII
GLUTEUS MEDIUS
TENSOR FASCIA LATAE
SEMIMEMBRANOSUS
VASTUS LATERALIS
ACHILLES TENDON

TRAPEZIUS
INFRASPINATUS
BICEPS BRACHII
LATISSIMUS DORSI
FOREARM FLEXORS
GLUTEUS MAXIMUS
ADDUCTOR MAGNUS
GRACILUS
SEMITENDINOSUS
BICEPS FEMORIS LONG HEAD
BICEPS FEMORIS SHORT HEAD
SARTORIUS
GASTROCNEMIUS
SOLEUS

Figure 7.1
STRUCTURAL DESIGN OF HUMAN SKELETAL MUSCLE.

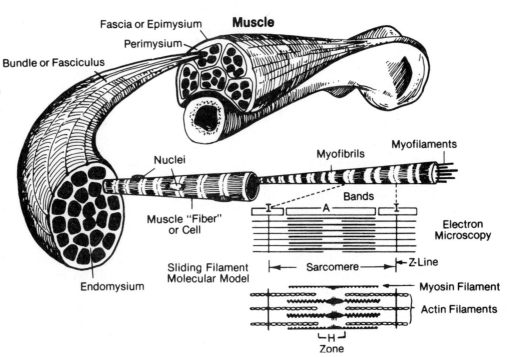

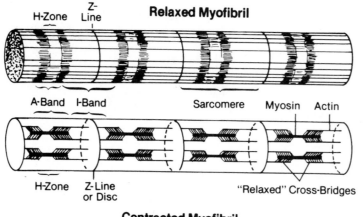

Relaxed Myofibril

H-Zone — Z-Line

A-Band I-Band — Sarcomere — Myosin Actin

H-Zone — Z-Line or Disc — "Relaxed" Cross-Bridges

Contracted Myofibril

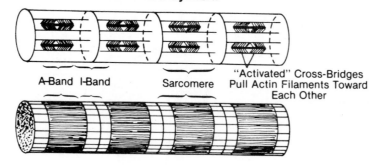

A-Band I-Band — Sarcomere — "Activated" Cross-Bridges Pull Actin Filaments Toward Each Other

Figure 7.2
THE SEQUENCE OF EVENTS THAT TAKES PLACE WITHIN A MYOFIBRIL DURING CONTRACTION.

From Jack H. Wilmore and David L. Costill, *Training for Sport and Activity,* 3d ed. Copyright © 1988 Wm. C. Brown Publishers, Dubuque, Iowa. All Rights Reserved. Reprinted by permission.

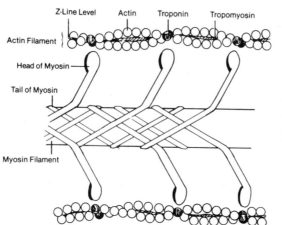

Z-Line Level — Actin — Troponin — Tropomyosin

Actin Filament

Head of Myosin

Tail of Myosin

Myosin Filament

Figure 7.3 MYOSIN MOLECULES HAVE PROJECTIONS THAT EXTEND TOWARD NEARBY ACTIN FILAMENTS.

From Jack H. Wilmore and David L. Costill, *Training for Sport and Activity,* 3d ed. Copyright © 1988 Wm. C. Brown Publishers, Dubuque, Iowa. All Rights Reserved. Reprinted by permission.

AGONIST AND ANTAGONIST

Muscles and muscle groups work in harmony to produce a movement. When the leg is extended, the muscle responsible for that movement is called the agonist or prime mover. Another muscle, the antagonist, has to relax to allow for smooth movement. In leg extension movements, the quadriceps are the agonists, and the hamstrings are the antagonists. The antagonists are also capable of resisting agonist action and are responsible for movement in the opposite direction. The antagonists of the prime mover that extends the leg are responsible for flexing it. If both agonists and antagonists contract at the same time, the part they act upon will remain stationary. Smooth coordinated movements depend upon the prime mover and antagonist working in harmony. It is therefore important to strengthen both groups of muscles and not one at the expense of the other.

11. In executing a half knee bend from an erect position, how does the force of gravity affect the actions of the agonist and antagonist muscle groups?

TENDONS

Tendons are the extension of the outer cover of the muscle and anchor the muscle to the bone. They have the appearance of white glistening cords or bands.

LIGAMENTS

Ligaments are strong flexible bands or capsules of fibrous tissue that help hold the bones together at the joints. They play a significant role in determining the range of motion of the joint.

ATROPHY

With a lack of neural stimulation and exercise, a wasting process may take place in which the muscle becomes smaller and weaker. This process, called atrophy, is often apparent when a limb has been in a cast or immobilized for an extended period of time.

SLOW- AND FAST-TWITCH MUSCLE FIBERS

Human muscles contain three types of muscle fibers: a slow-twitch Type I *red fiber* and two types of fast-twitch Type II *white fibers*. Each fiber type is structurally and chemically equipped to perform work for long or short periods of time. For example, fast-twitch fibers are preferentially used for short-term, high-intensity exercises such as sprinting, while slow-twitch fibers are used during longer, less intensive exercise such as long-distance running.

Exercise cannot change the types or numbers of fibers in your muscles, as these characteristics (or traits) are inherited. However, the efficiency of both red and white muscle fibers can be increased through proper training methods. A specific type of exercise must be used to improve the efficiency of a given fiber type. For example, to increase the metabolic potential of fast-twitch fibers, high intensity exercise of few repetitions must be used. Conversely, exercises of longer duration with lower intensities increase the metabolic potential of slow-twitch fibers.

Fast-twitch fibers produce greater force than slow-twitch fibers. As a result, individuals with a greater cross sectional area of fast-twitch fibers are capable of generating greater strength. Fast-twitch units, however, are quick to fatigue from very intense contractions, which demand high rates of force development.

HYPERTROPHY

Hypertrophy is an increase in the size and functional capacity of a muscle. There are two types of hypertrophy, transient and chronic. Transient hypertrophy is caused by the pumping action of the muscle and results in fluid accumulation in the muscle. This temporary enlargement disappears shortly after termination of exercise. In chronic (or true) hypertrophy the muscle growth results from enlargement of the muscle fiber. This growth is directly related to the increased synthesis of protein that increases the thickness of the myofibrils. Tension overload may also stimulate proliferation of connective tissue, capillarization, and satellite cells that surround the muscle fibers and improve the *structural integrity of ligaments and tendons*. The greatest hypertrophy is seen in those muscles that in everyday activity do the least work in relation to their genetic potential. The tension a muscle develops during exercise is a stimulus for increased uptake of amino acids and enhanced synthesis of protein. In addition, it is thought that a breakdown and buildup process takes place. This theory holds that intensive training breaks down muscle protein that then rebuilds between training sessions and leads to a super compensation and an increase in muscle size. However, the exact cellular mechanism by which resistance training results in increased muscle size is still unknown.

The degree of hypertrophy will depend not only on the severity of the overload but the total duration of the overload. However, one must be cautioned about individual exceptions to this principle. For instance, individuals with a large number of fibers may have an advantage in terms of their capacity for training over those with fewer fibers, particularly in body building. Also, evidence indicates that body builders who engage in high-volume, low-intensity training gain increased size of slow-twitch fibers and increased capillarization. Power lifters who engage in low-volume, high-intensity training gain increased size of fast-twitch fibers with decreased capillarization.

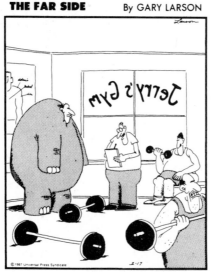

THE FAR SIDE By GARY LARSON

"I don't know what to tell you, Mr. Miller, but something has definitely gone awry with your workout program."

HYPERPLASIA

Hyperplasia is an increase in the number of muscle fibers. Considerable controversy still exists regarding whether or not heavy resistance training results in an increase in muscle fibers (hyperplasia). Recent research has criticized the methodology used in former studies that found some evidence of fiber splitting. The differences in research results may be due to differences in the mode of training as well as methodology. The consensus is that weight training or other exercises do not result in an increase in the number of muscle fibers; rather they increase the size and functional capacity of existing fibers.

12. What steps can be taken to limit or relieve the muscle soreness that usually is first felt twelve to forty-eight hours following vigorous exercise?

MUSCLE SORENESS

Many individuals engaged in rigorous exercise encounter muscle soreness. Two different patterns of soreness are apparent. The first type is soreness that occurs during the latter stages of, or immediately after, exercise. This type of soreness is thought to result from high hydrostatic pressure caused by fluid from the blood entering the muscle tissue. The second type of soreness generally appears twelve to forty-eight hours after a strenuous exercise. We have all had the unpleasant experience of waking up the next morning barely able to move after a previous day's exercise. This type of soreness is thought to be the result of small tears in muscle tissue or possible spasms in the muscle brought about by reduced blood supply. Generally muscle soreness after exercise can be limited if there is a good pre- and post-warm-up and stretching. Stretching can also bring some relief from existing pain in the muscle. Easy swimming or cycling can help reduce soreness.

Table 7.1

Weight Exercises and Major Muscles Involved

Biceps—Barbell curls, dumbbell curls, pull-ups, reverse curls.

Triceps—French curls, tricep extensor (standing or lat machine). Bar-dips, military press, bench press, pull-over (bent arm).

Brachialis—Reverse curls, upright rowing.

Deltoids—Military press, behind the neck press, dumbbell press, upright rowing, pull-overs (bent arm), lateral raise (standing), bent rowing.

Flexor carpi—Wrist curls, curls, grip machine.

Pectoralis—Bench press, lateral raise (incline or supine), pull-over and press, lat pull (machine).

Trapezius—Shoulder shrugs, behind the neck press.

Rhomboids—Bent rowing, shoulder shrugs, lat pull (machine).

Latissimus dorsi—Lat pull (machine), bent rowing, dumbbell rowing, pullover (bent arm).

Serratus—Pull-over (bent or straight arm).

Abdominals—Sit-ups (all varieties), scissor kick (incline), leg lifts (hanging), leg pullover (incline).

External obliques—Side bending (dumbbell or barbell), stiff-legged side lift.

Erector Spinae—Stiff-legged dead lift, dead lift, back hyperextensions.

Gluteus Maximus—Squats, leg press (machine).

Quadriceps—Squats, leg press (machine), knee extension (machine).

Hamstrings—Knee flexions (machine), squats.

Gastrocnemius and soleus—Toe raises (leg press machine or standing).

Glossary

Actin   Thin contractile protein in muscle fibers.
Agonist   Muscle responsible for movement.
Antagonist   Muscle that relaxes to allow agonist to contract.
Atrophy   Decrease in the size of muscle tissue.
Epimysium   Fibrous connective tissue surrounding skeletal muscle.
Fasciculus   Bundles of muscle fibers enclosed by connective tissue, which make up a skeletal muscle.
Fast Twitch   Fast-twitch Type II muscle fibers physiologically adapted for short-term, high-intensity exercise.
Hyperplasia   An increase in the number of muscle cells.
Hypertrophy   Enlargement in muscle size.
Ligament   Connective tissue that attaches bone to bone.
Muscle Soreness   Muscle pain resulting from chemical or physical changes in the muscle tissue.
Myosin   Thick contractile filaments that make up the muscle fibers.
Slow Twitch   Slow-twitch Type I muscle fibers physiologically adapted for endurance activity with a high capacity to use oxygen.
Tendon   A cord of connective tissue that attaches muscle to bone.

chapter 8

training concepts

Objectives

After studying this chapter you should be able to:

1. Define strength, power, and speed.

2. Describe force potential.

3. Describe nerve control of skeletal muscles.

4. Define isotonic, isometric, eccentric, concentric, and isokinetic contraction.

Strength training has finally emerged from the dark ages of ignorance and uncertainty. In recent years a great deal of excellent research has occurred in the areas of muscle cell physiology and muscle training techniques. As a result, a substantial body of knowledge has been established that supports a number of basic muscle training concepts.

STRENGTH, POWER, AND SPEED

There has always been a great deal of interest in the amount of maximal force or strength potential of muscles. *Muscle strength* (the amount of force that can be exerted by a muscle group for one movement or repetition) has always been considered to be an essential basis of athletic skill. Strength training by its nature emphasizes the force component of a movement but not the acceleration component essential in power. Recently, however, new interest has arisen in the maximal rate that a muscle can generate and transfer mechanical energy, which is expressed as power. Power is basically the product of strength and speed (power = force $\times$ distance/time). It is obvious from this formula that muscle power is dependent on the interaction of strength and speed. An increase in either force or speed will result in increased power. However, strength will play only a minor role unless the athlete can apply it explosively over a short period of time. The great majority of sports require power and, though strength is an essential ingredient of power, speed must receive special consideration. For example, the strongest football lineman may not necessarily be the best if he doesn't have the speed that allows him to outmaneuver and outleverage his opponent. The quickness of the first step in basketball, changing direction in football, and the explosiveness out of the starting blocks in sprinting also point out the critical interaction between muscle force and speed.

The effects of strength training on muscle speed are not well understood. However, speed training is different from strength training. Strength training requires a high level of resistance that prohibits fast movement. Speed, on the other hand, can best be enhanced by repeatedly practicing the specific movements required in the particular sport skill. Because speed depends upon activating the appropriate neuromuscular pattern involved in a particular skill, it is important to train at velocities of movement similar to or faster than those of the specific sport movement. Speed is defined as strength guided by skill. To increase speed, one needs to increase strength and to maintain or increase skill.

Another consideration sometimes overlooked when the emphasis is on strength is that high power efforts typically involve high movement velocities that are coupled with brief contraction time. In rapid movement there is little kinesthetic feedback to the individual regarding the amount of force generated. It is possible that many athletes who train with weights become conditioned to make their best efforts when they can sense the force they are developing. It is tempting to speculate that successful athletes may be those who have learned to use upper motor centers for performing maximum power contractions without relying on kinesthetic feedback or relying on a critical feedback period of short duration.

Strength

An enhanced arousal level and accompanying nerve disinhibition and/or possible neural facilitation are the probable explanations for the unexplained feats of strength performed in emergency situations. In such situations an individual is capable of achieving his or her individual maximum level of strength. Significant changes in neural facilitation also occur in the early stages of strength training programs, which partly account for rapid increases in strength in these stages.

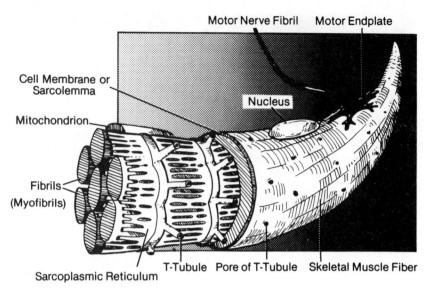

Nerve impulse transmission. From Jack H. Wilmore and David L. Costill, *Training for Sport and Activity*, 3d ed. Copyright © 1988 Wm. C. Brown Publishers, Dubuque, Iowa. All Rights Reserved. Reprinted by permission.

Neuromuscular Facilitation

A *motor unit* consists of a motor nerve cell (neuron) that originates in the spinal cord and all the muscle fibers supplied by that neuron. The number of muscle fibers innervated by a single motor nerve varies from a few in some eye muscles to as many as a thousand in the large thigh muscle. All of the muscle fibers within a given unit are of the same fiber type. The muscle fibers are located throughout the muscle and all contract simultaneously when stimulated by the nervous system. Even though patterns of motor unit activity are still not well understood, it is apparent that different patterns are optimal for different activities.

Force Potential

There are basically three ways in which training overload can enhance the maximal strength of muscles. These are: the number of motor units called into action, the frequency of the nerve impulses, and the coordination of nerve impulses. Increased frequency of nerve impulses results in increased force and decreased frequency in decreased force. The degree of muscle tension is dependent upon the number and frequency of motor units activated by the central nervous system. The more units recruited, the stronger the maximal contraction. Finally, nerve impulses have to be properly synchronized to allow for unified contraction, which is essential for maximum force.

Nerve Impulses and Strength

Both excitatory and inhibitory stimuli descend from the brain to the motor nerves. One explanation for increases in strength is that through training one can learn to decrease the inhibitory impulses from the brain to the muscles, thus allowing for a greater recruitment of force. In other words, physical training may be responsible for various adaptations of the brain and spinal cord. Another factor to consider is that certain muscle groups can be maximally activated through voluntary muscle contraction while others cannot. It may be that those muscles that can be more voluntarily activated receive greater stimulation from the brain. Unfortunately, evidence in this area is somewhat incomplete.

Muscle Cross Section

One of the best indicators of the maximum strength capability of a muscle is its cross sectional area. The larger the cross section, the greater the potential strength of the muscle and vice versa. This fact is particularly true in isolated muscles where there is an extremely high correlation between cross sectional area and maximal force. However, the relationship is much less in the whole organism than in the isolated muscle. Also, it has been found that increases in strength as a result of training may sometimes be disproportionate to muscle size and due possibly to improved neural facilitation. This observation may explain why women are able to make significant increases in strength with small changes in cross sectional muscle size.

Muscle Length

There is an optimum length of a muscle at which it can generate its greatest force. Muscles are generally their strongest at a length slightly longer than their normal resting length in their fully extended position. Muscles are weaker at shorter and longer lengths than the optimum.

Weight Resistance Methods

As a general rule, a muscle worked close to its maximum capacity will increase in strength. The overload can be applied by a wide variety of weight lifting equipment, free weights, ropes, isokinetic devices, pulleys, and so on. Strength improvement is governed primarily by the intensity of the overload and not the method, though certain methods may be more appropriate in some circumstances than others. Isotonics, isometrics, eccentric, and isokinetic contractions are the most widely used techniques for increasing strength and endurance in muscles.

MUSCLE CONTRACTION

Isotonic Exercise

Isotonic exercise is exercise that is performed against resistance while the load remains constant. The resistance varies with the angle of the joint, for example, lifting free weights (barbells) or weight stacks, such as those used in the universal gym. Free weights are most popular among today's athletes as they feel that the motions are most similar to sport skill movements.

Eccentric Loading

Eccentric loading is sometimes referred to as a negative contraction because the muscle lengthens as it develops tension. An example would be letting yourself down slowly from a chin-up. This type of exercise tends to produce more muscle soreness, possibly due to micro tears in the muscle fibers and tendons, than other techniques. It is not superior to other isotonic methods but is used mainly as a supplement to other training techniques.

Isometric Exercise

An isometric exercise is a contraction performed against a fixed or immovable resistance, where tension is developed in the muscle, but there is no change in the length of the muscle or the angle of the joint. Isometric exercise is also called static contraction. An example would be holding a heavy weight in one position for a fixed amount of time or pushing against a wall.

It appears that with isometric exercise strength development is specific only to the joint angle stimulated during training. As a result, isometric exercise does not increase strength throughout the range of movement. Isometric exercise also may inhibit the ability of the muscle to exert force rapidly, such as is necessary in the shot put and discus events. In addition, isometric exercise increases pressure in the chest cavity, which results in reduced blood flow to the heart, lungs, and brain, along with increased blood pressure. Consequently, isometric exercises are not recommended for individuals with cardiovascular problems. There also may be some decrease in muscular endurance as isometrics restricts peripheral blood flow during the static contraction.

Isokinetic Exercise

An isokinetic exercise is a contraction in which the muscle contracts maximally at a constant speed over a full range of the joint movement against a variable resistance. Isokinetic means equal motion, which is interpreted to mean equal rate of motion or equal speed. An isokinetic contraction can be accomplished only with the use of special equipment, such as a minigym that utilizes "accommodating resistance." In other words, the harder you pull, the harder the gym resists you—the resistance is always related to the applied force.

Unlike with other types of resistance training in isokinetic exercise, there is no set resistance to meet. Rather the velocity of movement is controlled. The resistance offered by the machine cannot be accelerated and any force applied against the equipment results in equal reaction of force. This makes it possible for a person to exert maximum effort throughout the full range of movement. Another advantage is that isokinetic equipment allows one to approximate the same force and same velocity as that encountered in athletic competition. Isokinetic resistance also provides a safer alternative to other exercise programs, especially during the process of muscle rehabilitation. Isokinetic exercise may also be used to quantify a muscle group's ability to generate torque or force, and is also useful as an exercise modality in the restoration of a muscle group's pre-injury level of strength.

When training isokinetically, it is necessary to exert as much force against the resistance as possible for maximal strength gains to occur. It is easy to "cheat" and not go through the workout at high intensity. Cheating may be hindered if there is a partner around to supply motivation.

High-velocity training is not as specific as slow exercise training in bringing about strength gains. Training at fast velocities tends to increase strength at and below the exercise velocity. Exercise at slow velocities tends to produce strength increases specific to training velocities.

It is apparent that many combinations of sets and repetitions of isokinetic training will result in increases in strength. Examples of isokinetic equipment are the Cybex, Lido, Mirac, Biodex, Kincom, and Orthotron.

Isokinetic exercise has become popular because it provides a speed-specific indication of the absolute strength of the muscle group being trained, thus enabling one to more closely replicate some specific athletic skills. The most effective strength gains have come from speeds of approximately sixty degrees (measure of distance) per one second or less. Recent research, however, has indicated that training at fast speeds of movement generally increases strength at all speeds of movement.

13. What is the primary training factor governing the degree of improvement in the strength of a muscle?

ADVANTAGES AND DISADVANTAGES OF WEIGHT-RESISTANCE PROGRAMS

Isotonic, isometric, eccentric, and isokinetic exercise all have their advantages and disadvantages. As long as the muscle is overloaded, however, it will gain in strength.

Isotonic Exercise

Advantages

1. It generally produces strength gains throughout the full range of movement.
2. Progress in strength gains is easy to evaluate because of numbered free weights and universal stacks.
3. Strength exercises can be developed to duplicate a variety of sports skills.
4. If free weights are used, balance and symmetry are enhanced.

Disadvantages

1. The equipment is cumbersome.
2. There is a greater potential for accidents.
3. Most strength gains occur at the weakest point of the movement and are not uniform throughout.

Eccentric Exercise

Advantages

1. It is as effective in strength gains as isotonic and isometric exercise.
2. It increases motivation of some individuals who enjoy lifting heavier resistance.
3. It may increase one's skill by lowering resistance slowly.
4. It can duplicate a variety of movements.

Disadvantages

1. It can cause greater post-exercise soreness than other methods.
2. A partner as spotter is needed to lift heavier resistance.

Isometric Exercise

Advantages

1. Little time is required for training.
2. Expensive and cumbersome equipment is not needed.
3. Exercise can be performed anywhere—in home, office, or on vacation.

Disadvantages

1. Strength gains are not produced throughout the full range of movement.
2. Strength gains are difficult to evaluate; that is, no numbered weights or gauges are customarily used.
3. It increases the pressure in the chest cavity, causing reduced blood flow to the heart, lungs, and brain.
4. It is not as efficient in producing strength gains as isotonic and isokinetic methods.
5. It is not effective in producing increases in skilled movements.
6. Motivation is difficult to maintain.
7. Muscular endurance may decrease.

Isokinetic Exercise

Advantages

1. It produces maximum resistance through the full range of movement.
2. It increases strength throughout the full range of movement.
3. It may result in less injury and soreness than isometric and isotonic exercise.
4. The uniqueness of the equipment may increase motivation.
5. Strength gains are easy to determine.
6. It is adaptable to specific movement patterns.
7. It permits skill improvement.

Disadvantages

1. The equipment is very expensive, with limited availability.
2. Research is still incomplete with regard to motor patterns and force-velocity relationships.

3. Applicability to sport-specific ballistic skills may be limited and may be best for tension skills (e.g., swimming and running).
4. A high level of motivation is required to give full effort to each exercise.

Glossary

Eccentric   Exercise in which the muscle lengthens as it develops tension.

Isokinetic   A contraction in which the muscle contracts maximally at a constant speed over a full range of joint movement against a variable resistance.

Isometric   A contraction performed against a fixed or immovable resistance where tension is developed in the muscle, but there is no change in the length of the muscle or angle of the joint.

Isotonic   Exercise against resistance while the load remains constant, with the resistance varying with the angle of the joint.

Muscle Strength   The amount of force that can be exerted by a muscle group for one movement or repetition.

Power   The product of strength and speed.

Speed   Strength guided by skill.

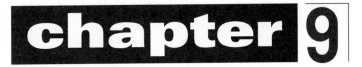

advanced training

Objectives

After studying this chapter you should be able to:

1. Describe the pyramid system.
2. Describe single sets.
3. Describe the multi-poundage system.
4. Describe the super pump system.
5. Describe super sets.
6. Describe burnouts.
7. Describe partial repetition.
8. Describe circuit training.
9. Describe periodization.
10. Describe forced repetition.
11. Describe negative work.
12. Describe split routine.
13. Describe plyometrics.

Once you have mastered the basic techniques of strength training and have developed a high level of strength and endurance, you may be tempted to enter into advanced training.

No unanimity of opinion exists on the best training system, but generally success in weight training will depend on your progression and quality of work.

The following systems and techniques are commonly used today by advanced weight lifters. Optimal gains, strength, and hypertrophy can be achieved by mixing various training programs and manipulating the training variables.

PYRAMID SYSTEM

The pyramid system is the most popular system for strength and power development. Progression from a low weight to a higher weight with a decreasing number of repetitions is the hallmark of this system. Following is an example of a pyramid system:

Table 9.1

	Pyramid System	
Set Number	**Number of Repetitions**	**Weight (in lbs)**
1	10	155
2	8	185
3	6	205
4	4	225
5	2	245
6	1	255

The athlete may then work his way back down to lower weights and higher repetitions.

SINGLE SET SYSTEMS

Single set systems consist of the performance of one set of each exercise, eight to twelve repetitions. These are not as efficient in producing strength and endurance gains as multiple sets.

MULTI-POUNDAGE SYSTEM

The multi-poundage system requires the assistance of one or two spotters. The individual performs 4 to 5 RMs. Then the spotter removes twenty to forty pounds from the bar. The individual then performs four to five more repetitions, and continues this procedure for several sets. The number of sets depends upon the original resistance used. This program is used primarily to increase muscular endurance.

SUPER PUMP SYSTEM

The super pump system is primarily for body builders. The individual starts off with fifteen to eighteen sets for each body part and one to three exercises for each muscle group per training session. There is a fifteen-second rest period between sets of five to six repetitions. These exercises are useful primarily for the large muscles in the arms, chest, and shoulders.

SUPER SETS

In the super set system the lifter performs one exercise and quickly follows it with another exercise, then rests. The individual works on the two exercises alternately until a desired number of sets has been completed. Adding a third exercise to this routine is called trisets.

BURNOUTS

In the burnout system, after you complete what is normally your last set, you take some weight off the bar and immediately do an additional set. You continue doing sets with less weight each time and without rest for up to five or six sets or until exhaustion.

PARTIAL REPETITIONS

At the end of the last repetition, usually of the last set of an exercise, when the lifter is unable to perform another full repetition, he or she performs one-half, one-third, or one-fourth of a repetition until these cannot be continued.

FORCED REPETITION

After the last full repetition of the last set, the spotter helps the lifter perform another one to three repetitions by assisting the lifter as needed to complete the repetitions.

NEGATIVE WORK

After the last set has been completed, additional weight is added to the bar and the lifter with the aid of spotters slowly lowers the weight. The spotters then raise the weight and the lifter lowers it again. This process may be repeated for three to five repetitions and several sets.

SPLIT ROUTINE

Rather than performing the entire workout program in one day, many lifters break up their programs into alternate day routines. A lifter may work the upper body on Monday, Wednesday, and Friday, and the lower body on Tuesday, Thursday, and Saturday. This routine results in more workouts per week but each workout is shorter. Many athletes find that they can perform higher intensity workouts with this method.

PLYOMETRICS

Plyometrics are exercises in which the muscle is loaded suddenly and forced to stretch before the contraction of movement occurs. The greater the stretch put on the muscle from its resting length immediately before the concentric contraction, the greater the resistance the muscle can overcome. Plyometrics emphasize the speed of the eccentric phase. The rate of stretch is more critical than the magnitude of stretch. These exercises were developed to enable the muscle to reach maximum strength in as short a time as possible. Examples include jumping off a box onto the ground and rebounding as quickly as possible. The deceleration and acceleration of body weight provides the overload. Upper body plyometrics include medicine ball throws, catches, and several types of push-ups.

Plyometric exercises are beneficial in sports that require the application of maximal force during high speed movements, sometimes referred to as speed-strength. The individual should be well into a strength training program before attempting plyometrics. Refer to table 9.2 for plyometric intensity levels, and to figure 17.1 for plyometric exercise machine.

Definitions of Plyometric Exercises

Jump—A movement that concludes with a two-foot landing.
Jump in place—Vertical jump performed in place (tuck, pike, split squat, squat, power jumps).
Standing jump—A maximal jump that may be linear, vertical, or lateral.
Hop—A move that starts and concludes with a one-foot or two-foot landing of the same foot or feet (short hop, ten repetitions; long hop, thirty repetitions or more).
Bound—Series of movements in which one lands successfully on alternate feet (short-response bound, twenty-five–thirty meters; long-response bound, sixty meters or more).
Shock—In-depth jump and box jumps (few use this method).

Caution—This combination of high force and speed produces very significant loads on the muscles, tendons, and ligaments. These structures need to be well conditioned to both force and speed before plyometric exercises are attempted. Proper technique and form are very important in performing these exercises in order to reduce the impact shock and to protect the joints and joint structure.

PERIODIZATION

The underlying principle of periodization is related to Hans Selye's general adaptation syndrome. Selye's theory states that there are three phases of the body's adaptation when it is confronted with a stress stimulus, in this case, resistance training. The first phase is termed the shock or alarm phase, which lasts one to two weeks. Soreness and stiffness may develop, with a slight decrease in performance. In the second phase,

Table 9.2

Plyometric Drills, Classified by Intensity Level			
	Low intensity	**Medium intensity**	**High intensity**	**Shock**
In-place jumps	• Squat jump • Split squat jump • Cycled split squat jump (Also: ankle bounce, ice skater, lateral cone jump)	• Pike jump • Double-leg tuck jump (Also: Jump-up, lateral hop)	• Double-leg vertical power jump • Single-leg vertical power jump • Single-leg tuck jump	
Standing jumps		• Standing triple jump (Also: Standing long jump)		
Short-response hops		• Double- and single-leg zigzag hop and double-leg hop	• Single-leg hop and double- and single-leg speed hop	
Long-response hops		• Double-leg hop	• Single-leg hop and double and single-leg speed hop	
Short-response bounds		• Alternate leg bound • Combination bound		
Long-response bounds		• Alternate leg bound • Combination bound		
Shocks				• In-depth jump • Box jump
Upper body plyometrics	• Medicine ball sit-up • Plyometric sit-up (Also: two-hand overhead forward throw, clap push-ups)	• Medicine ball push-up (Also: overhead backward throw, underhand forward throw, Russian twist)		• Drop-and-catch push-up

adaptation to the training and performance demands increases. This phase is sometimes called super-compensation. The third phase is staleness, for the body no longer adapts to the new stimulus, which results in overwork, staleness, and exhaustion.

The key to periodization is to reduce the risk of overtraining and subsequent staleness and keep the exercise stimulus effective in order to maintain a high level of performance.

Periodization consists of four phases in each training cycle, not including active rest. The overall training period is referred to as a macrocycle, which may range from three months to four or five years. Within the macrocycle are two or more mesocycles consisting of a few weeks to a few months. Each mesocycle is broken down to a number of microcycles of about a week in length. A mesocycle is made up of three periods: preparatory, competition, and transitional.

Following a season of competition is a period of transition, which includes active rest for a period of one to four weeks. During this time the individual may participate in a variety of leisure sports activities. Only low-volume and light resistance training should be engaged in during this time of recovery from the stress of competition.

The preparatory phase that follows the transition phase includes a hypertrophy phase, strength phase, power phase, and peaking phase. The hypertrophy phase consists of high-volume, low-intensity exercise, three to five sets of eight to twelve repetitions, fifty to seventy-five percent, 1 RM. The strength phase consists of moderate volume and increased intensity, three to five sets of five to six repetitions, eighty to eighty-eight percent, 1 RM. The power phase consists of low-volume, high-intensity exercise, the major goal being to bring about increases in maximum strength, three to five sets, two to four repetitions, ninety to ninety-five percent (high intensity), 1 RM. The peaking phase consists of very low volume and high intensity, where the goal is to peak strength for a particular competition, one to three sets, one to three repetitions, one hundred percent, 1 RM.

Periodization can be used also for cardiorespiratory training. It consists of gradually reducing volume while increasing intensity to accomplish specific sports requirements. The concept of periodization with its four phases makes it possible to develop a resistance training program for any sport.

STRENGTH AND POWER

Hypertrophy	3–5 sets	8–20 RM
Strength	3–5 sets	2–6 RM
Power	3–5 sets	2–3 RM
Peaking	1–3 sets	1–3 RM

It is vital to understand how to manipulate intensity and volume for specific sports. Variation in training is essential to maintain motivation and reduce monotony and boredom.

Most sports have a schedule that includes an off-season, preseason and an in-season period.

Off-season—Period between last contest and six to eighteen weeks prior to first contest.

Preseason—Six to eight weeks prior to first contest.

Competitive period—All contests scheduled for that season.

The majority of athletes today use some kind of cycling in their training. By manipulating the load and frequency of exercise, the volume of exercise can be controlled. Training cycles may progress from high volume/low intensity to low volume/high intensity. This gives the body time to recover and adjust to training demands while still allowing for a maximal exercise stimulus; the body is able to meet the high demands encountered during competition. (See appendix H for examples of training cycles.)

Examples of Cycles

4 weeks	10 RM	3–4 days a week
4 weeks	8 RM	4 days a week
4 weeks	4 RM	5 days a week
4 weeks	1–3 RM	6 days a week

Another option is to vary the number of weeks for each different training load.

3 weeks	10–12 RM
7 weeks	8 RM
4 weeks	3 RM
2 weeks	1–3 RM

It is extremely difficult to maintain a peak level of fitness for more than a few weeks during the in-season. It is important to develop a training cycle that peaks the individual for the most important contest. Low volume and greater intensity are essential for the most critical events.

Table 9.3

Typical Training Mesocycle for a Sprinter

Season designation	Period/phase designation	Training schedule
Off-season	**Preparatory period** • **Hypertrophy/endurance phase**	*Flexibility training:* ballistic, static, or proprioceptive neuromuscular facilitation (PNF) stretching *Resistance training:* specific or nonspecific exercises of high volume and low intensity *Metabolic training:* aerobic activities *Speed training:* high-volume, low-intensity technique training
	Transition (optional) • **Strength phase**	All training of low volume and low intensity *Flexibility training:* ballistic, static, or PNF *Resistance training:* specific exercises of moderate volume and intensity *Metabolic training:* interval work *Speed training:* moderate-volume and moderate-intensity technique training, including towing and downhill activities
Preseason	• **Power phase**	*Flexibility training:* ballistic, static, or PNF stretching *Resistance training:* specific exercises of low volume and high intensity *Metabolic training:* short work intervals of maximal and near-maximal intensity with full recovery intervals *Speed training:* high-intensity, low-volume activities
	Transition period (optional)	All training of low volume and low intensity
In-season	**Competition period**	*Flexibility training:* ballistic, static, or PNF stretching All training of low volume and high intensity *Resistance training:* low-volume, high-intensity, sport-specific exercises *Metabolic training:* race-specific intervals with full or near-full recovery between intervals
Off-season	**Transition period**	*Optional:* recreational games; light, unsupervised training

From Dan Wathan, Periodization, concepts and applications, in *Essentials of Strength Training and Conditioning,* ed. Thomas Baechle. Champaign, IL: Human Kinetics, 1994.

Glossary

Burnout   Continued sets with reduction in resistance until exhaustion.

Circuit Training   A combination of strength and/or endurance exercises performed in sequence at various stations.

Forced Repetitions   Performing additional repetitions with assistance when muscle can no longer complete movement.

Multi-Poundage System   Progressive reduction in training load.

Negative Work   Exercise in which spotters raise the weight, lifter slowly lowers the weight.

Partial Repetition   Performing an exercise without moving the weight through the complete range of motion at either the beginning of a repetition or at the end of a repetition.

Periodization   Calendar year broken down into various training cycles.

Pyramid System   Progression from low weight to higher weight with decreasing number of repetitions.

Plyometrics   Exercise in which the muscle is loaded suddenly and forced to stretch before the contraction for movement occurs.

Single Set   The performance of one set for each exercise.

Split Routine   A routine in which certain parts of body are worked on one day and other parts on alternate days.

Super Sets   Alternating back and forth between two exercises until the prescribed number of sets are completed.

Super Pump System   Fifteen to eighteen sets for each body part. And one to three exercises for each muscle group.

chapter 10

exercises

Objectives

After studying this chapter you should be able to:

1. Describe a strength exercise for the chest.
2. Describe a strength exercise for the back.
3. Describe a strength exercise for the shoulder.
4. Describe a strength exercise for the trunk.
5. Describe a strength exercise for the hips.
6. Describe a strength exercise for the thighs.
7. Describe a strength exercise for the calf muscles.

This chapter provides a selection of the most effective and popular exercises for various body parts. (See figures 10.1 through 10.33.) These include exercises with free weights and machines. The section includes weight training exercises for chest, back, shoulder, arms (biceps, triceps, and forearms), trunk (abdominals and lower back), hips, and thigh and calf.

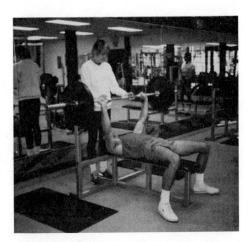 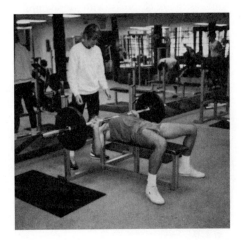

Figure 10.1 BENCH PRESS.

Muscles Used:

Primary: *Pectoralis Major.*
Additional: *Anterior Deltoid, Biceps Brachii, Triceps Brachii.*

The weight is lowered to the chest and returned to the starting position. Hands are slightly wider than shoulder width; thumbs should be wrapped around the bar, with feet flat on floor.

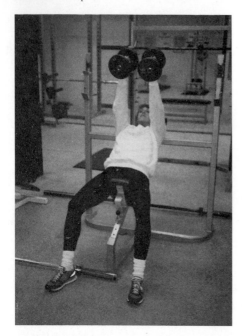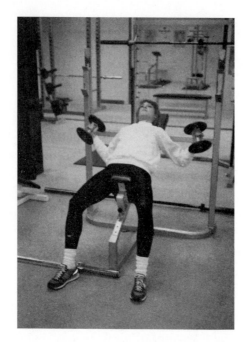

Figure 10.2 INCLINED DUMBBELL FLY.

Muscles Used:

Same as in bench press, with more emphasis on the upper Pectoralis Major fibers.

Lower the dumbbells to the side with a wide elbow position, then return to starting position.

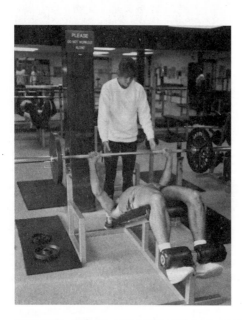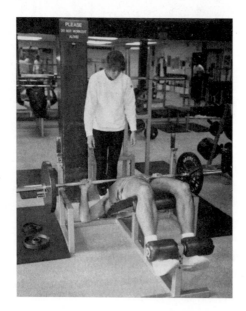

Figure 10.3 DECLINED BENCH PRESS.

Muscles Used:

Primary: *Same as in bench press but with more emphasis on lower portion of Pectoralis Major.*

The weight is lowered to the chest and returned to the starting position. Hands are slightly wider than shoulder width; thumbs should be wrapped around the bar, with feet flat on floor.

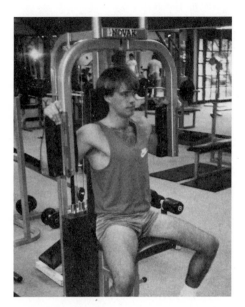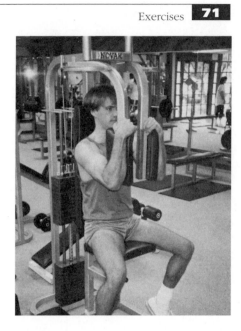

Figure 10.4 PEC DECK MACHINE.

Muscles Used:

Pectoralis Major with emphasis on the inner/medial fibers.

From the starting position bring your arms together until the machine arms nearly touch, then return to starting position.

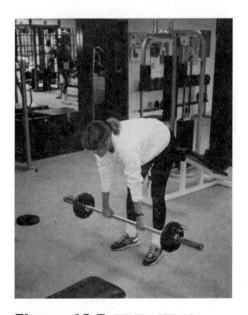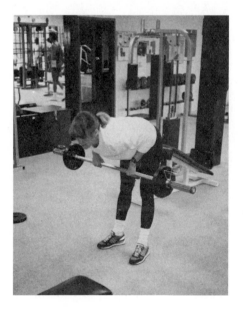

Figure 10.5 BENT ROWING.

Muscles Used:

Primary: *Upper back musculature, Rhomboid Major and Minor, Teres Major and Minor.*
Additional: *Posterior Deltoid Latissimus Dorsi.*

Place feet shoulder-width apart. Hands should be about shoulder-width apart with knees slightly bent. The bar is lifted to the chest and then lowered. Be careful not to twist or jerk the lower back. The exercise can be done with the head resting on a bench or table to help support the lower back.

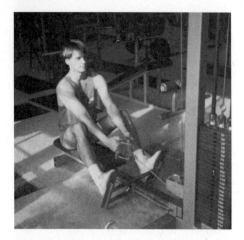
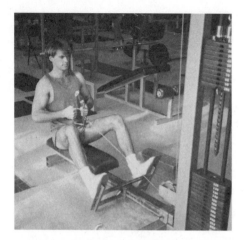

Figure 10.6 SEATED PULLEY ROWS.

Muscles Used:

Same muscles as in bent rowing.

Knees are bent and the back is held straight. The hand grip is brought to the chest and then returned to the starting position.

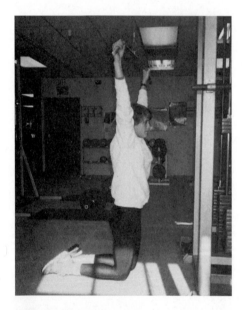
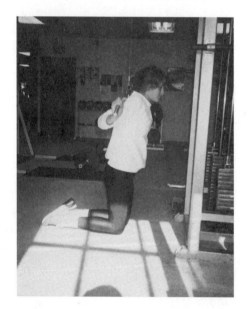

Figure 10.7 LATERAL PULL DOWN.

Muscles Used:

Latissimus Dorsi.

A wide grip is taken on the bar and then the bar is pulled to shoulder level. For heavy resistance, a seated position can be used to enable a restraining bar to be placed above the knees in order to keep the body down.

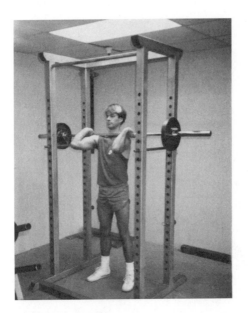
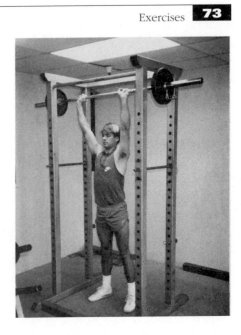

Figure 10.8 PRESS (MILITARY PRESS).

Muscles Used:

Primary: *Trapezius, Deltoid.*
Additional: *Supraspinatus, Levator Scapulae.*

Feet are placed flat on the floor approximately shoulder-width apart. The hand grip is slightly wider than shoulder-width. The bar is pressed overhead and then returned to the starting position.

In figure 10.8 a weight rack is used that provides a safety measure for heavy weights. When lifting high resistances in this lift, a weight belt may be used to support the lower back.

If a weight rack is not used, the weight is brought from a floor resting position up to the on-shoulder position in what is called a clean movement.

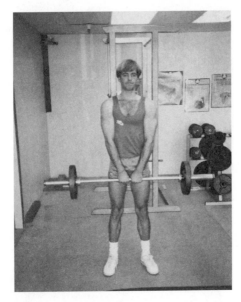
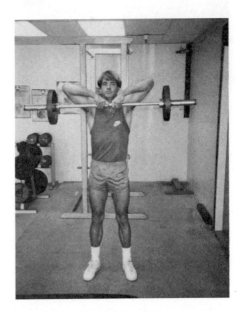

Figure 10.9 UPRIGHT ROWING.

Muscles Used:

Primary: *Trapezius, Deltoid.*
Additional: *Supraspinatus, Levator Scapulae.*

A close, narrow grip is used. The bar is brought up to just below chin level and returned to the starting position.

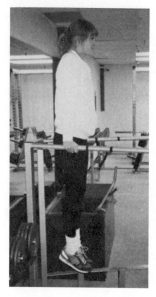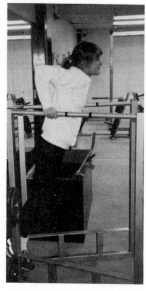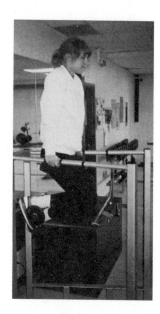

Figure 10.10 SHOULDER DIPS.

Muscles Used:

Primary: *Anterior Deltoid Pectoralis Major.*
Additional: *Triceps Brachii, Biceps Brachii.*

This exercise is performed on parallel bars. From the upright position, lower yourself to as low a position as possible, then push up to the upright position. The exercise may be performed with weights held by the feet and legs (see fig. 10.10).

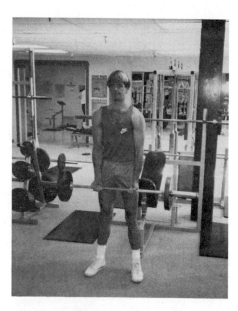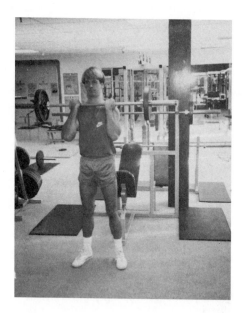

Figure 10.11 CURL.

Muscles Used:

Primary: *Biceps Brachii, Brachialis.*
Additional: *Coracobrachialis, Brachioradialis, Anterior Deltoid.*

Feet and hands shoulder width apart. The bar is brought up to the shoulders and returned to the starting position. Keep your back straight and knees slightly bent to discourage cheating.

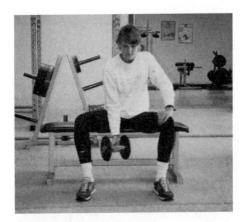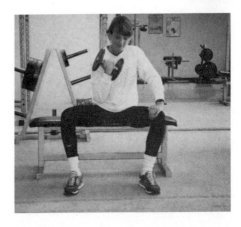

Figure 10.12 SEATED ALTERNATE DUMBBELL CURLS.
Muscles Used:

Same as in curl.

Seated position with feet and knees wide apart. The elbow of the lifting arm is in tight to the thigh. The opposite hand rests on the opposite thigh. After the target number of repetitions is achieved, the weight is switched to the other hand.

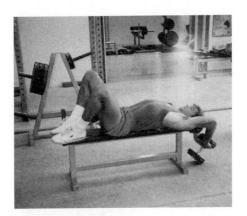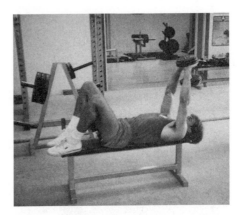

Figure 10.13 TRICEP PULLOVERS.
Muscles Used:

Primary: *Triceps Brachii.*
Additional: *Pectoralis Major, Latissimus Dorsi.*

This exercise is especially effective for working the long head of the Triceps.

Lie on a bench with the feet on the bench or flat on the floor. Hold the dumbbell with both hands and bring it up from the floor to a position directly above the head. Return it to near the floor.

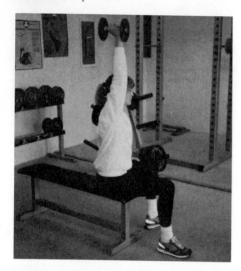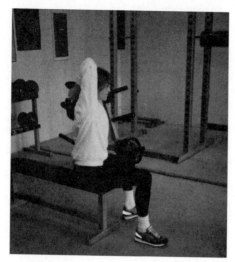

Figure 10.14 SEATED TRICEPS DUMBBELL CURLS.
Muscles Used:

Primary: *Triceps Brachii.*
Additional: *Deltoid.*

From a seated position, using one arm at a time, bring the dumbbell down to a position between the shoulder blades (scapulae) and return to the starting position.

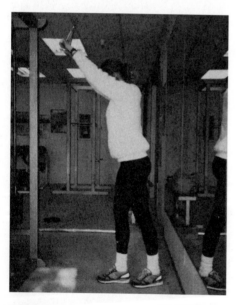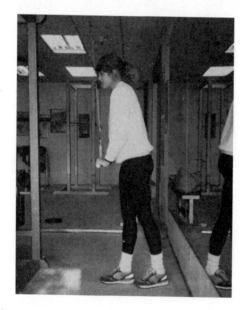

Figure 10.15 TRICEP PULLDOWNS.
Muscles Used:

Primary: *Triceps Brachii.*
Additional: *Posterior Deltoid, Latissimus Dorsi.*

Use a narrow grip. Bring the bar down close to the body to a position in front of the hips with the arms fully extended. Be careful of using the trunk in an effort to handle more weight.

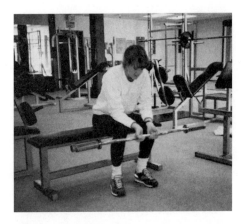 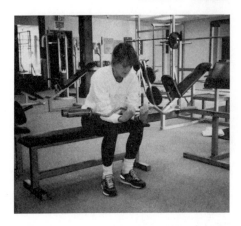

Figure 10.16 FOREARM CURLS.

Muscles Used:

Primary: *Forearm Flexors, Flexor Carpi Radialis, Flexor Carpi Ulnaris.*
Additional: *Flexor Digitorum Profundus, Flexor Digitorum Superficialis.*

Rest the forearms on the thighs for support. Hold the bar with a palm-up grip, and flex the hands and wrist upwards. A reverse, palm-down grip can be used to perform a reversed forearm curl for development of the posterior forearm muscles.

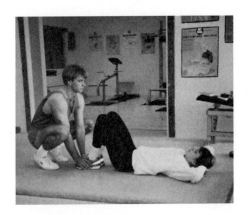 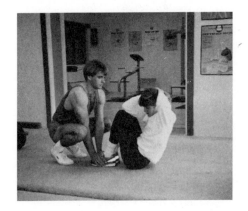

Figure 10.17 BENT-KNEE SIT-UPS.

Muscles Used:

Primary: *Rectus Abdominis.*
Additional: *Internal Obliques, External Obliques, Transverse Abdominis.*

Start flat on the floor with feet secured under a dresser, pads, or sit-up board. A spotter also can hold your feet. Bend knees to at least a ninety degree angle to place less stress on the lower back. Straight-up sit-ups work primarily the rectus abdominis while twisting sit-ups add work for the oblique muscles.

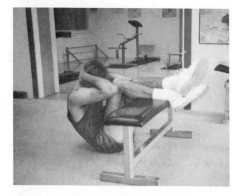

Figure 10.18 CRUNCHES.

Muscles Used:

Same as in bent-knee sit-ups.

Place legs on a bench. Start this sit-up flat on the floor and bring torso up until elbows touch the knees.

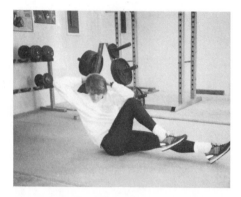

Figure 10.19 ALTERNATE KNEE TOUCHING SIT-UPS.

Muscles Used:

Abdominal Group.

Starting flat on the floor, raise upward and touch your elbow to your opposite knee. Repeat for the opposite elbow and knee. This exercise is excellent for oblique development.

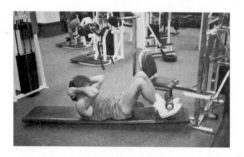

a.

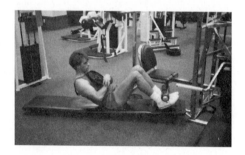

b.

Figure 10.20 (*a*) SIT-UPS ON AN INCLINE BENCH.

(*b*) SIT-UPS WITH WEIGHTS.

Muscles Used:

Abdominal Group.

Start flat on the floor and move to a fully trunk upright position.

The use of weights adds resistance for greater strength development.

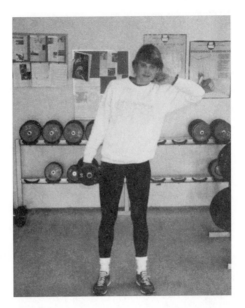 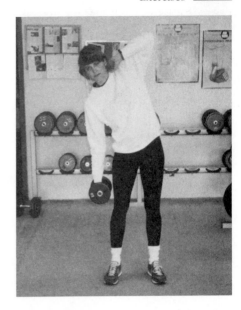

Figure 10.21 SIDE BEND WITH DUMBBELL.

Muscles Used:

Primary: *Transverse Abdominis.*
Additional: *Internal Obliques, External Obliques.*

From an upright standing position, bend to the side, stretching the opposite side. Try to concentrate on isolating the musculature to slowly return to the upright position.

Be careful not to use too heavy a weight as this area will increase in size.

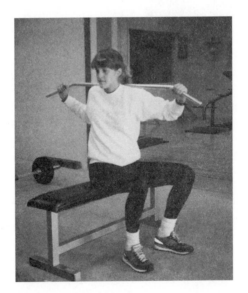 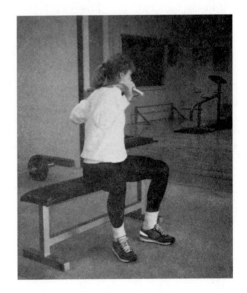

Figure 10.22 SEATED BAR TWISTS.

Muscles Used:

Primary: *Transverse Abdominis.*
Additional: *Internal Oblique, External Oblique.*

From a seated or standing position with a bar or broomstick on your shoulders and your hands spread wide and grasping the bar, twist to one side and reverse twist to the other.

Try to isolate the abdominal muscles while performing this exercise.

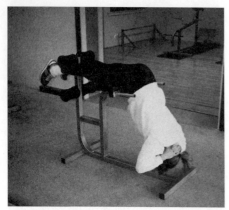

a.

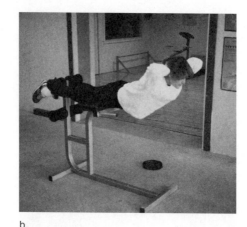

b.

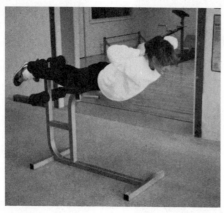

c.

Figure 10.23 (*a* & *b*) BACK HYPEREXTENSION (*c*) WITH WEIGHTS.

Muscles Used:

Primary: *Erector Spinal Group.*

Using a back hyperextension machine, start from the down (flexed) position and move upward into a hyperextended position. This exercise can be performed with light weights to build greater strength. Take care, however, as the lower back muscles are subject to spasms. Use only light weights.

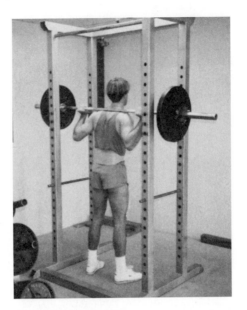

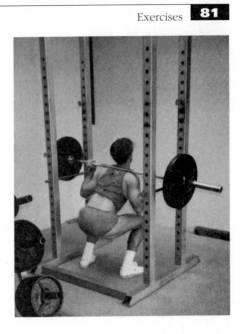

Figure 10.24 (*a* & *b*) HALF SQUAT.

Muscles Used:

Primary: *Gluteals, Quadriceps, Hamstrings.*

The safest way to perform squats is to use a squat rack, as shown in figure 10.24. Starting from an upright position with the bar on your shoulders, bend at the knees and slightly lower yourself to a position of a ninety degree angle between your thigh and leg. This is a half squat. Full squats put great stress on the knees and can produce injuries in susceptible individuals. We recommend half squats.

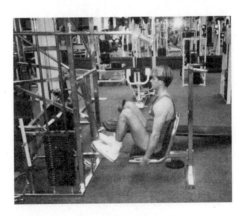

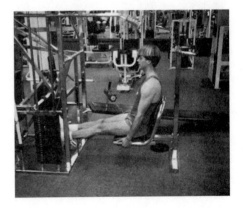

Figure 10.25 LEG PRESS.

Muscles Used:

Primary: *Quadriceps.*
Additional: *Hamstrings, Gluteals.*

Adjust the seat so that there is a ninety degree angle or less at the knees. From this position press until legs are extended.

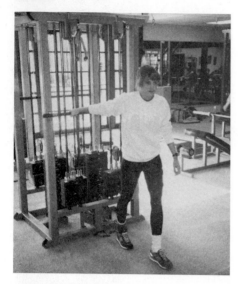
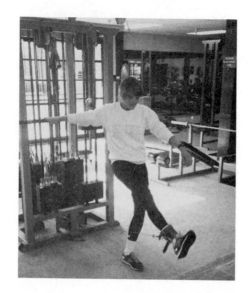

Figure 10.26 HIP FLEXION.

Muscles Used:

Primary: *Ileopsoas.*
Additional: *Rectus Femoris, Quadriceps Group.*

Face away from the weight pulley. Extend your leg behind you, then bring the leg forward.

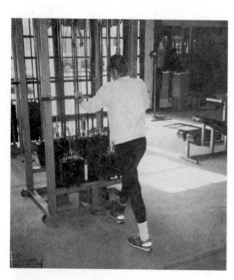
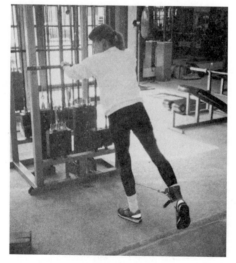

Figure 10.27 FOUR-WAY HIP EXTENSION.

Muscles Used:

Primary: *Gluteals.*
Additional: *Hamstrings.*

Place your leg in front of you, then bring your leg backwards into a hyperextended position behind you.

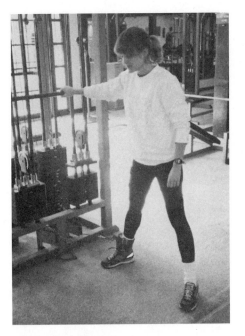
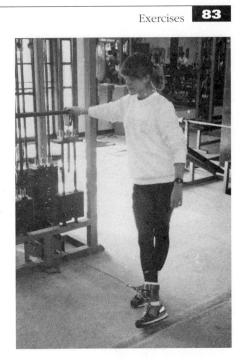

Figure 10.28 HIP ADDUCTION.
Muscles Used:

Primary: *Adductor Group.*
(Groin Muscles)

Stand with legs wide apart, then bring one leg inward and across in front of the support leg.

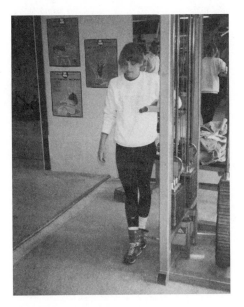
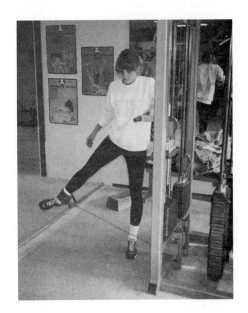

Figure 10.29 HIP ABDUCTION.
Muscles Used:

Primary: *Gluteus Medius, and Minimus.*
Additional: *Tensor Fascia Latae.*

From a position slightly in front of the support leg, move the leg outward to the side.

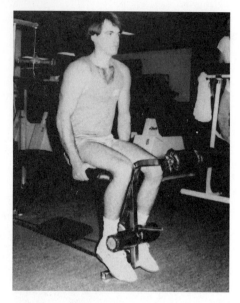 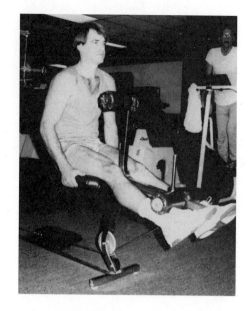

Figure 10.30 LEG EXTENSION.

Muscles Used:

Quadriceps.

Move the legs from a flex position to an extended position, pause momentarily, and return. Start with your legs at a right angle and pause with your legs straight.

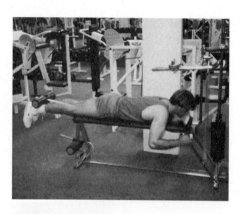 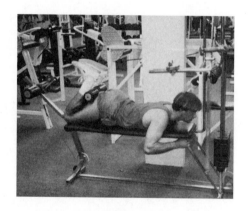

Figure 10.31 LEG FLEXION.

Muscles Used:

Primary: *Hamstrings (Semitendinosus, Semimembrinosus, Biceps Femoris).*

Lying prone on the bench with your heels behind the pads, flex the legs and bring your heels toward your buttocks.

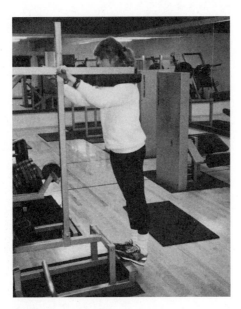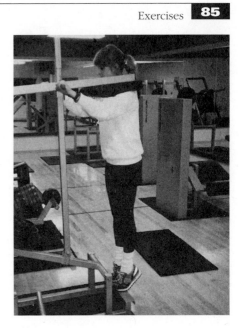

Figure 10.32 TOE RAISE.

Muscles Used:

Primary: *Posterior Calf groups, Gastrocnemius, Soleus.*
Additional: *Tibialis Posterior.*

Starting from a position in which your heels are lower than your forefeet, press upwards using the calf muscles until you are standing on your toes.

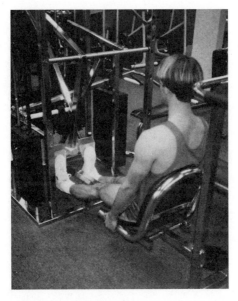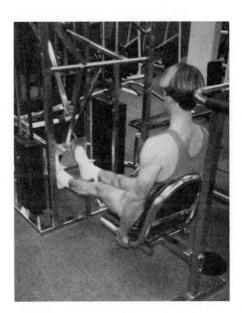

Figure 10.33 SEATED TOE RAISES.

Muscles Used:

Same as in toe raise.

Slide your feet halfway down the foot platform so that the balls of your feet are on the platform but your heels are off. Press forward and back from a toes-back to a toes-forward position.

chapter 11

women and weight training

Objectives

After studying this chapter you should be able to:

1. Describe the effect of strength training on women.

2. Describe the physical differences between men and women that are significant in strength training.

3. Define amenorrhea.

4. Describe exercise guidelines for pregnancy.

Female participation in physical activities has increased markedly over the past few years as outdated social mores regarding women's involvement in exercise and sport have changed.

Increasingly, more and more women are lifting weights. To those of us who have enjoyed the benefits of weight training, the increase in women's weight training is not at all surprising. Having known the benefits for years, we realized that as women began to lift they too would enjoy and desire the benefits of weight training.

One reason why the increase has been so dramatic is that women have found that through weight training they have become stronger. Being stronger improves your confidence, your self-image, and your concept of what goals can be achieved. In few, if any, athletic endeavors are these experiences so quickly enjoyed, dramatic in effect, and repeatedly reinforced.

Let's look at some special training considerations for women and their impact on weight training.

PHYSIOLOGY

Men's and women's response to cardiorespiratory training is nearly identical. When it comes to skeletal-muscular training, however, some differences in response to training do occur. These differences are not a function of muscle physiology but rather hormonal influences.

Women have a smaller amount of muscle mass and greater amount of subcutaneous fat stores that tend to lessen muscle definition. Women on average have about three-quarters the amount of absolute strength of males; however, their percentage of strength increases as a result of training is approximately the same. Also, female body builders have dramatically high lean to fat ratios in comparison with other female athletes.

Males have a much higher level of testosterone circulating within their bodies. This male sex hormone is also present in women but in significantly less amounts. The influence of testosterone on skeletal muscles is, with the aid of training, to increase muscle mass. Because women have lower levels of testosterone, the increase in muscle mass (hypertrophy) that they experience with weight training is significantly less. Very few women increase dramatically in muscle mass as a result of weight training. Those that do may have an unusually high level of testosterone in their systems or may be using anabolic steroids (see chapter 16).

Most women respond to weight training by increasing their strength, endurance, and muscle tone, but they do so without the significant increases in muscle mass that men experience. Very few women need to worry about becoming "too big" or "masculinized" as a result of weight training. However, with exceptional overload and volume they may increase muscle mass.

If a woman chooses to use anabolic steroids to raise her testosterone level, she will respond to training in the same manner as a man and will produce muscle mass increases in a similar fashion. There are, however, side effects to using anabolic steroids that may be unacceptable to her, such as deepening voice, increase in body hair, acne, high blood pressure, and other problems (see chapter 16).

Men, on the other hand, exceed women in maximum oxygen consumption during exercise. This is believed to be due to greater cardiac output, blood volume, and oxygen-carrying capacity of the blood. Also, because men have more lean muscle in relation to total body weight than women, they have about thirty to forty percent greater absolute strength. Their overall stores of energy-rich compounds, such as ATP, PC, and glycogen, also are greater.

Women's response to physical training in terms of cardiorespiratory endurance, muscle metabolism, and strength however, is similar to that of men.

PHYSICAL DIFFERENCES

The bone structure of the female pelvic girdle is wider than a male's to facilitate the birthing process. Women's knees, however, are approximately the same distance apart as a man's. This combination results in a greater convergence angle and stress, and, thus, a greater likelihood that women will experience knee problems when performing squats, particularly deep or full squats. Women should gradually increase the resistance they use in these lifts to prevent this problem.

Percentage of Body Fat

Women have a higher percentage of body fat than men. This is true in the general population (men, twelve to seventeen percent; women, nineteen to twenty-four percent) as well as in comparing male and female athletes (men, four to ten percent; women, ten to fourteen percent). Exercise can reduce body fat, and this reduction occurs without sex discrimination. Women often, however, start with a higher percentage and retain a higher percentage even when highly trained (as compared to a highly trained male).

Menstruation

The cause of exercise amenorrhea (cessation of menstruation) is still unknown. However, a number of theories exist, including increased testosterone and decreased ovarian function, loss of body fat, and active pituitary functioning. Presently, there is a strong indication that a change in hypothalamic functioning may be responsible. Sufficient calcium replacement is essential for individuals encountering amenorrhea.

Most women who cease menstruation appear to suffer no physiological problems, but the long-term effects are unknown. If amenorrhea does occur, cutting back on training, eliminating stress, and raising the percentage of body fat above ten percent are recommended.

EXERCISE GUIDELINES FOR PREGNANCY

14. Exercise in moderation, and particularly rhythmic activity, is recommended for pregnant women within appropriate guidelines. Which specific types of movement are counterindicated?

1. Exercise intensity should not go beyond the seventy percent threshold level. The American College of Obstetricians and Gynecologists cautions against heart rates exceeding 140 beats per minute.
2. Exercise should be stopped if there is any pain or bleeding.
3. Adequate intakes of iron, calcium, and vitamins should be insured before and during pregnancy.
4. Avoid bouncing, jarring, and twisting activities that put your abdomen in jeopardy.
5. If you feel tired or experience discomfort, stop and rest.
6. You should not exercise so intensely that you are unable to talk.
7. Don't exercise while lying on your back after the fourth month. This can block the blood supply to the uterus and depress fetal heart rate. If you need to rest, lie on your side.
8. Don't exercise vigorously in hot weather (core body temperature should not go above 101 degrees Fahrenheit).
9. Drink plenty of water before, during, and after exercise.
10. Your exercise program should be started well in advance of your pregnancy.
11. Research is not confirmed regarding the detrimental effects of a pregnant mother being involved in such activities as gymnastics and yoga.

If a pregnant woman has medical problems, disease, or other complications, she should seek advice from an obstetrician before undertaking a rigorous physical exercise program. Rhythmic, moderate activity is well advised and safe for both mother and fetus.

EXERCISE AFTER CHILDBIRTH

Women who have just given birth should start exercising as soon as possible if there were no complications and if they have received medical clearance from their physician. They should start slowly because their red blood cell count may be a little low, resulting in feelings of fatigue and shortness of breath. Gradually, over four to six weeks, they should be able to work up to the exercise routine they maintained before they became pregnant. If, during exercise, they feel themselves getting overly tired, they shouldn't force themselves to complete the exercise. Moderation is the key until their bodies start responding and they feel as though they can exercise without undue stress.

OSTEOPOROSIS

Osteoporosis is a disease in which bone tissue degenerates. It ranks closely behind arthritis as a major chronic disease of older people, especially women. Susceptibility to the disease appears to increase with menopause. It may be that the estrogen decreases that accompany menopause hasten the destruction of bone tissue and also decrease the body's absorption rate of calcium, which is vital for the integrity of the bones.

There is a wide variation in bone density among women. Physical activity, calcium intake throughout life, ability to adapt to low-calcium diets, and fluoride intake are all associated with higher bone density. On the other hand, a lack of regular menstruation, premature menopause, use of some medications, and prolonged bed rest are associated with low bone density. It is important, therefore, not to focus attention on calcium alone when a number of factors play a significant part in this disease. Evidence from the National Institute of Health indicates that taking calcium supplements after menopause has only a marginal effect on bone loss. The NIH recommends that all adults consume 1,000 milligrams of calcium daily, and post-menopausal women who are considered to be at high risk for the development of osteoporosis should consume an additional 500 milligrams.

Some success has resulted from a combination of increased calcium intake with an aerobic exercise program. Weight training with light weights supplemented with the proper diet may prove to be an answer, as training has been shown to increase bone density in all age groups regardless of gender.

15. Calcium is one factor controlling the degree of bone density. What other factors have been identified as influential?

Glossary

Amenorrhea   Abnormal cessation of menstruation.

Anabolic Steroids   Synthetic hormones that are similar to the male hormone testosterone.

Hypothalamus   Portion of brain controlling hormonal functioning among many other responsibilities.

Menopause   The natural cessation of menstruation occurring near age fifty.

Osteoporosis   A loss in bone materials and density, producing brittleness and softness of the bone.

chapter 12

cardiorespiratory fitness

Objectives

After studying this chapter you should be able to:

1. Describe cardiorespiratory fitness.
2. Describe the target heart rate method.
3. Define aerobic and anaerobic exercise.
4. Describe intensity, duration, and frequency of cardiorespiratory training.
5. Define cooling down.
6. Describe the American College of Sports Medicine Recommendations about Exercise.
7. Describe pre-exercise screening.

The body's ability to deliver oxygen and nutrients rapidly and efficiently to all vital organs such as the heart, nervous system, and working muscles is the basis of cardiorespiratory endurance. A well-conditioned heart and efficient respiratory system are essential to a high level of physical fitness. Table 12.1 lists the benefits of cardiorespiratory training on the body.

MAXIMUM OXYGEN UPTAKE

The main function of the heart and circulatory system is to provide blood, which is necessary to maintain the proper functioning of all body cells. In terms of exercise, the heart's main concern is its ability to deliver oxygen to the working cells of the body and to rid the cells of waste products. The greatest amount of oxygen used by the cells during maximum exercise per unit of time is referred to as **maximum oxygen uptake.** Maximum oxygen uptake is one of the best indexes of cardiorespiratory fitness. Training may be a twenty percent contributing factor in determining maximum oxygen uptake, whereas the remaining eighty percent is thought to be genetically determined.

The amount of blood pumped out per beat **(stroke volume)** at rest for the average individual is approximately 70 to 90 milliliters. During rigorous activity, the average heart may pump 100 to 120 milliliters per beat. The trained individual, however, may have a stroke volume at rest of 100 to 120 milliliters and a maximum capability during exercise of 150 to 170 milliliters. This gives the trained individual a decided advantage, since the more efficient your heart, the greater its ability to maintain exercise levels for long periods of time with less stress. The hearts of some trained individuals may be capable of pumping out as much as 30 to 35 *liters* a minute. This amount is six times the total volume of the blood in the body, which indicates the truly exceptional efficiency of the heart.

CARDIORESPIRATORY ENDURANCE

Cardiorespiratory endurance is the body's ability to sustain prolonged vigorous exercise. Muscular endurance, though partly dependent on the cardiorespiratory system, refers to the ability of a muscle or muscle group to sustain prolonged movement. Muscular endurance is related to muscular strength and is specific to the muscles that are being exercised.

Table 12.1

Benefits of Cardiorespiratory Training		
Cardiorespiratory Training Increases	Cardiorespiratory Training Produces	Cardiorespiratory Training Decreases
Tolerance to stress	Lower resting heart rate	Obesity-adiposity
Arterial oxygen content	Physical conditioning of muscles	Arterial blood pressure
Electron transport activity	Greater oxygen utilization	Heart rate
Efficiency of the heart	Greater stroke volume	Vulnerability to dysrhythmias
Blood vessel size		Stress response
Efficiency of blood circulation	Lower heart rate for submaximal work	Need of heart muscle for oxygen

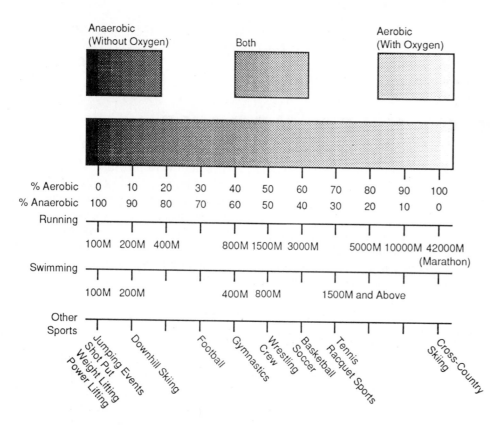

Figure 12.1 RELATIVE AMOUNTS OF ANAEROBIC VERSUS AEROBIC FITNESS REQUIRED IN DIFFERENT SPORT ACTIVITIES.

From *Aerobic Weight Training* by Frederick C. Hatfield, Ph.D. Copyright © 1985 Contemporary Books, Inc. Reprinted by permission of Contemporary Books, Inc.

In the running and swimming events, researchers generally agree that at around three minutes (until about seven or eight minutes) there are relatively equal requirements in both the aerobic and annaerobic pathways for muscle energetics.

AEROBIC-ANAEROBIC

All-out exercises lasting two minutes or less without stopping are referred to as anaerobic exercises (without oxygen). Such exercises as sprinting, tennis, handball, and weight lifting are examples of anaerobic exercises. For all-around physical fitness anaerobic exercise should be accompanied by continuous vigorous exercise lasting beyond two minutes, such as jogging, cycling, and swimming, which train the aerobic system (with oxygen). It is important to do aerobic training before participating in anaerobic activities such as strength training.

Figure 12.1 shows the relative amounts of aerobic versus anaerobic fitness required in different sport activities.

ENERGY SYSTEMS

The first energy source involves two energy-rich compounds—**ATP (adenosine triphosphate)** and **PC (phosphocreatine)**—that are stored directly in the muscle tissue. When the muscle is stimulated through exercise, ATP and PC break down and release immediate energy for muscle contraction. Energy from ATP and PC, however, is available only for a brief period because only very small amounts of these compounds are stored in the muscle. This concept is known as **anaerobic** (without oxygen).

A second energy source during exercise is supported by sugar, which is stored in the muscles in the form of glycogen. When glycogen is broken down, the released energy produces more ATP. However, when glycogen is burned in the absence of oxygen, it gives off an end product called lactic acid, which results in muscle fatigue. For this reason, this energy source is limited to activities that last approximately one to two minutes. If exercise continues beyond this time, the body is required to draw upon oxygen, the third energy source available during exercise.

The oxygen system can use both glycogen and fats as fuel for the production of ATP. Lactic acid, along with the accumulation of calcium 2+ (ions) and heat, are major factors in muscle fatigue. However, when oxygen is used through a complex process that occurs in the muscle cells, the oxygen prevents the buildup of lactic acid and promotes the resynthesis of ATP for energy. This system is referred to as **aerobic** (with oxygen) and is used primarily in endurance activities, such as long-distance running, skiing, and swimming.

INTENSITY

16. Describe the principles that can ensure good cardiovascular training effects.

For a training effect to occur in the cardiovascular and muscular system, the exercise program must consist of activities that produce an overload on these systems. For cardiovascular training the threshold level is seventy percent of your maximum heart rate, as previously outlined. A threshold level of sixty percent is used for post-heart attack victims, obese persons, or persons with a history of sedentary living.

TRAINING EFFECT

Monitoring your heart rate is a very effective way of determining exercise intensity. This approach is referred to as the threshold effect or training heart rate effect. Research by Karvonen found that a training level of seventy percent of your maximum heart rate, approximately sixty percent of your maximum oxygen uptake level, is considered to be a minimal level of intensity necessary to increase cardiovascular endurance.

Determining your target heart rate is relatively simple. First you determine your maximum heart rate by subtracting your age from 220. This method is not an exact measure because the formula predicts rather than assesses. As a result, there is a possibility of a ten beat per minute error. Next, subtract your resting pulse rate from your predicted maximum heart rate, then multiply the difference by seventy percent. Add this product to your resting heart rate; the result will give you your target heart rate level. The resting heart rate is determined by taking your pulse in the morning before you get out of bed. Because of daily fluctuations you should average this figure for three to five days.

The following is an example of determining the target heart rate level for a twenty-year-old individual with a resting heart rate of seventy beats per minute:

220 − 20 = 200 beats per minute (maximum heart rate) where 20 is the individual's age.
200 − 70 = 130 (70 is the resting heart rate in this example)
130 × .70 = 91 (.70 is the desired intensity)
91 + 70 = 161 beats per minute where 70 is the resting heart rate

The target heart rate level in this example is 161 beats per minute.

Table 12.2

Approximate Energy Cost (in Kilocalories) of Various Physical Activities	
Sport or Activity	**Kilocalories Expended per Minute (kcal/min) of Activity**
Climbing	10.7–13.2
Cycling 5.5 MPH	4.5
9.4 MPH	7.0
13.1 MPH	11.1
Dancing	3.3–7.7
Football	8.9
Golf	5.0
Gymnastics	
Balancing	2.5
Abdominal exercises	3.0
Trunk bending	3.5
Arm swinging, hopping	6.5
Rowing 51 str/min	4.1
87 str/min	7.0
97 str/min	11.2
Running	
Short distance	13.3–16.6
Cross-country	10.6
Tennis	7.1
Skating (fast)	11.5
Skiing, moderate speed	10.8–15.9
Uphill, maximum speed	18.6
Squash	10.2
Swimming	
Backstroke	11.0
Breaststroke	11.5
Crawl (55 yd/min)	14.0
Wrestling	14.2

Source: Reprinted by permission of the American Alliance for Health, Physical Education, Recreation and Dance, 1900 Association Drive, Reston, Virginia 22091.

Three basic principles are important to insure proper cardiovascular training effects: intensity, duration, and frequency.

Also refer to tables 12.2 and 12.3 which relate energy to type and intensity of exercise.

DURATION

How long you exercise depends primarily on the intensity of the exercise and your long-range goals. Beginners should exercise for a minimum of fifteen to twenty minutes. As fitness level improves, the exercise session can be increased from thirty to sixty minutes. Maintaining your target training effect level during the thirty to sixty minutes of exercise will improve your cardiorespiratory endurance. Longer work periods are necessary only for those interested in competing in such activities as long-distance running

Table 12.3

Typical Criteria for the Classification of Exercise Intensity

Exercise Intensity Classification	Criteria Heart Rate	Energy Expenditure (kcal/hr)	Perceived Exertion
Very light	<110	<110	Very, very easy
Light	110–120	111–270	Easy, no pain or discomfort
Moderate	121–150	270–400	Somewhat difficult and slight discomfort
Heavy	151–160	401–550	Difficult, uncomfortable, and some pain
Very heavy	161–180	550–669	Very difficult and painful
Exhaustive	>180	>700	Extremely difficult and painful

Source: From Hage, Phillip, "Perceived Exertion: One Measure of Exercise Intensity," in *The Physician and Sports Medicine*, September 1981, pp. 136–46. © 1981 McGraw-Hill Healthcare Group. Reprinted by permission.

or swimming. Strength training should be approximately fifteen minutes in duration. Generally, longer exercise sessions over thirty-five minutes produce greater fitness benefits. However, low-fit individuals should start out with five- to ten-minute sessions equivalent to approximately 100 kilocalories per session and work up to expenditures of 200 to 300 kilocalories per workout. (A kilocalorie is the amount of heat necessary to raise one kilogram of water one degree Celsius.) Longer duration exercises tend to improve the muscle's ability to use fat. Presently there is no evidence to indicate that additional health benefits are derived from workouts that exceed 60 minutes (600 kilocalories). Therefore it is recommended that low-fit individuals' exercise should last long enough to burn 100 to 200 kilocalories; medium-fit, 200 to 400; and high-fit individuals, 400 or more kilocalories. There is considerable evidence now to indicate that exercise needs to exceed 7.5 kilocalories a minute to reduce the risk of heart disease.

FREQUENCY

You don't have to knock yourself out seven days a week to achieve cardiorespiratory endurance. Workouts three to five days a week are sufficient. It is important to allow yourself twenty-four to forty-eight hours for rest and recovery between exercise bouts.

Overstressing the body is one of the worst things you can do, and one way to do that is by strenuously exercising only once a week. This kind of regimen is worse than no exercise at all. Strenuous exercising once a week can greatly stress your cardiorespiratory system without producing any benefits. If you cannot exercise at least three times a week, then your once- or twice-a-week exercise should be moderate, with the main objectives of relaxation and burning up a few extra calories. In addition it may lower the risk of coronary heart disease.

Another thing to keep in mind is that if you miss a day or two in your exercise routine, you should never try to make it up. This is a dangerous practice, especially for middle-aged people. The important consideration here is not to become obsessive about exercising. Some people, whose main goal in exercising is to avoid having a heart attack, become so rigidly goal-directed that any interference in their exercise schedule results in anxiety. This is not the object of exercise. Your exercise program

Table 12.4

Stage	Duration	Activity
Warm-up, flexibility	10–15 minutes	Walking, slow jogging
Aerobic exercise	20–40 minutes	Bicycling,
		Walking,
		Jogging,
		Swimming
Cool down	8–10 minutes	Walking, stretching

Sequence and Time Ranges for Basic Fitness Program

should be enjoyable and relaxing. Avoid rigidly structured schedules that lead to anxiety and tension. And remember, don't "pile it on" if you miss a day.

These three workouts should be spaced evenly through the week to avoid long periods of nonactivity. A typical schedule is as follows:

3-day schedule
RUN M–W–F

5-day schedule
RUN M–W–F   or   RUN T–Th–Sat
BIKE T–Th   BIKE Sun–F

7-day schedule
RUN M–W–F
BIKE T–Th–Sat
SWIM Sun

COOLING DOWN

You should continue to exercise at a low intensity (stretching and walking eight to ten minutes) following a rigorous workout. (See table 12.4.) This step will allow your body to adjust to a resting state. Cooling down prevents the blood from pooling in the lower extremities, which could reduce the amount of blood returning to the heart and disrupt the cardiac cycle. Cooling down also helps reduce muscle soreness, dizziness, and the amount of biochemical fatigue products in the blood.

CIRCUIT TRAINING

Circuit training involves a combination of strength and endurance exercises performed in sequence at various exercise stations. This extremely efficient technique can be specifically designed for a variety of different sports activities. For example, the circuit can emphasize strength, muscular endurance, cardiovascular activities, or a combination of all three. Table 12.5 presents an example of a muscular strength, muscular endurance, and cardiovascular circuit training program. See appendix C for the Universal super circuit.

PRE-EXERCISE SCREENING

For many years in the United States, physicians adopted a somewhat restricted approach to exercise prescription, suggesting that a stress electrocardiogram was needed in all men over the age of thirty-five years who wanted to increase their habitual physical

Table 12.5

Muscle Strength and Cardiovascular Circuit-Training Program	
Duration	Ten weeks
Frequency	Three days per week
Circuits/session	Circuit A: 3; Circuit B: 2
Time/circuit	Circuit A: 7 1/2 min; Circuit B: 15 min
Total time/session	Circuit A: 22 1/2 min; Circuit B: 30 min
Load	40 to 55 percent of 1 RM
Repetitions	As many as possible in thirty seconds
Rest	Fifteen seconds between stations

Muscle Strength and Endurance Circuit A		Cardiovascular Circuit B	
Station	Exercise	Station	Exercise
1	Bench press	1	Running (440 yd)
2	Bent-knee sit-ups	2	Push-ups or pull-ups
3	Knee (leg) extension	3	Bent-knee sit-ups
4	Pulldown-lateral machine	4	Vertical jumps
5	Back hyperextension	5	Standing (overhead) press
6	Standing (overhead) press	6	Bicycling (3 min)
7	Dead lift	7	Hip stretch
8	Arm curl	8	Rope jumping (1 min)
9	Leg curl (knee flexion)	9	Bent-over rowing
10	Upright rowing	10	Hamstring stretch
		11	Upright rowing
		12	Running (660 yd)

Source: *Sports Psychology*, by Edward L. Fox. Copyright © 1979 by Saunders College Publishing/Holt Rinehart and Winston. Reprinted by permission of CBS College Publishing.

activity. This requirement has now largely been discredited. The need for extensive preliminary screening is particularly questionable given that modern exercise decreases rather than increases a person's overall risk of cardiac death.

The Canadian Physical Activity Readiness Questionnaire (rPAR-Q) (table 12.6) has proved to be a very safe screening and has shown remarkable success in detecting potential contraindications to exercise. The rPAR-Q is thus the currently recommended method of determining exercise readiness in symptom-free adults with no more than one major cardiac risk factor. A yes answer on one or more of the seven questions indicates the need for medical screening prior to beginning an exercise program.

EXERCISE PRESCRIPTION

17. Can you determine your target heart rate level by following the directions in the text?

The American College of Sports Medicine makes the following recommendations for the quantity and quality of training for developing and maintaining cardiorespiratory fitness and body composition in the healthy adult:

1. Frequency of training: three to five days per week.
2. Intensity of training: sixty percent to ninety percent of maximum heart rate.

Table 12.6

Suggested Lab Activity—Revised Physical Activity Readiness Questionnaire (rPAR-Q)

Yes	No	
____	____	1. Has a doctor said that you have a heart condition and recommended only medically supervised activity?
____	____	2. Do you have chest pain brought on by physical activity?
____	____	3. Have you developed chest pain in the past month?
____	____	4. Do you tend to lose consciousness or fall over as a result of dizziness?
____	____	5. Do you have a bone or joint that could be aggravated by the proposed physical activity?
____	____	6. Has a doctor ever recommended medication for your blood pressure or a heart condition?
____	____	7. Are you aware through your own experience, or a doctor's advice, of any other physical reason against your exercising without medical supervision?

NOTE: If you have a temporary illness, such as a common cold, or are not feeling well at this time—POSTPONE.

Produced by the British Columbia Ministry of Health and the Department of National Health and Welfare.

3. Duration of training: fifteen to sixty minutes of continuous aerobic activity. Duration is dependent on the intensity of the activity; thus lower intensity activity should be conducted over a longer period of time. Because of the importance of the total fitness effect and the fact that it is more readily attained in longer duration programs, and because of the potential hazards and compliance problems associated with high intensity activity, lower to moderate intensity activity of longer duration is recommended for the nonathletic adult.

4. Mode of activity: Any activity that uses large muscle groups, that can be maintained continuously, and is rhythmical and aerobic in nature: for example, running, jogging, walking, hiking, swimming, skating, bicycling, rowing, cross-country skiing, rope skipping, and various endurance game activities. See also figures 17.2–17.9 for cardiorespiratory machines.

EXERCISE PRECAUTIONS

Be familiar with the following exercise precautions before beginning your cardiorespiratory endurance program:

1. Get a thorough physical examination before starting your conditioning program.
2. If fatigue lasts two hours or more following an exercise session, the program is too rigorous. Reduce your level of exercise.
3. Alcohol and exercise do not mix. Alcohol constricts the coronary vessels of the heart muscle.
4. Cigarette smoking limits oxygen exchange in the lungs, thus preventing a high level of fitness attainment.
5. Always warm up before exercise and cool down after the activity.
6. Remember to use your heart rate as a guide to the intensity of the exercise.
7. Sporadic exercise may be detrimental to your health. Three to five exercise sessions a week are minimal for optimum benefit.

If any of the following symptoms occur while you are exercising, stop exercising and consult a physician before continuing your exercise program:

1. Fluttering, palpitating, missed, or extra heartbeats, sudden bursts of rapid heartbeats, or a sudden slowing of rapid pulse
2. Pressure or pain in the center of the chest, left arm, fingers, or throat
3. Dizziness, fainting, nausea, cold sweat, or light-headedness
4. Shortness of breath or inability to attain sufficient oxygen

Glossary

Aerobic   Continuous vigorous exercise of long duration, such as jogging, long-distance swimming, and cycling that utilizes large amounts of oxygen.

Anaerobic   All-out exercise lasting one to two minutes or less, such as weight lifting, sprinting, handball, and squash, performed in the absence of oxygen.

Cooling Down   Continuation of exercise at a low intensity following a vigorous workout, which allows the body to adjust to a resting state.

Duration   Amount of time utilized for each exercise bout.

Frequency   Number of exercise bouts per week.

Intensity   The level of physiological stress on the body during exercise.

Target Heart Rate   The proper intensity level of an endurance training program, approximately seventy to eighty-five percent of maximum heart rate.

chapter 13

flexibility

Objectives
After studying this chapter you should be able to:

1. Describe the importance of flexibility.
2. Differentiate between static stretching and ballistic stretching.
3. Describe the importance of stretching.
4. Describe PNF stretching.
5. Describe and demonstrate basic stretching exercises.

FLEXIBILITY

The term *flexibility* encompasses the ability to move freely throughout a full, nonrestricted, pain-free range of motion about a joint or series of joints. Flexibility is not only an important component of physical fitness but also is an important aspect of your resistance training program. There is a great deal of individual variation in joint looseness. Joint looseness may be the result of particular joint physical structure or unique individual characteristics.

Joint flexibility is controlled by a number of factors: the joint capsule contributes approximately forty-seven percent to the range of motion, the muscles contribute forty-one percent, the tendons contribute ten percent, and the skin contributes two percent. Because the joint capsule itself is rigid, the emphasis when attempting to increase or decrease flexibility is placed on the muscle and skin tissue. Stretching exercises enable these tissues to increase the range of the movement. Conversely, strengthening exercises may tighten up the muscles and tendons and can decrease the range of movement if not done correctly through the full range of motion.*

Women tend to have a greater range of movement in the joints than men primarily because men have generally larger and bulkier skeletal muscles, which tend to reduce joint movement. However, flexibility is one characteristic of well-developed muscles, regardless of gender.

All activities require varying degrees of flexibility. A competitive tennis player needs good shoulder flexibility. A laborer requires good lower-back flexibility. Even such everyday movements as walking and running require flexibility. Good flexibility reduces the possibility of the aches, pains, and inflammations associated with joints that are stressed through rigorous activity. Running for a long period of time without pre- and post stretching activities may lead to reduced flexibility in the legs and back and may result in lower-back problems.

There exists an erroneous concept that resistance training will result in a decrease of flexibility. Evidence indicates little support for this contention. Typically, heavy resistance training results in either an improvement or no change in flexibility. Care should be taken to stress the full range of motion of both agonist and antagonist muscle groups and to choose exercises that stimulate both groups of muscles at each joint to insure adequate strength and balance between both sides of the joints.

*Certain flexibility exercises have a greater potential for injury; therefore, caution should be observed when performing such exercises. Proper instruction by a certified professional in an exercise class is recommended if there is any doubt about a specific stretching exercise.

STATIC STRETCHING

Static stretching consists of stretching the muscle slowly and gradually for periods of ten to twenty seconds, followed by several seconds of relaxation. This method is a very effective stretching technique and does not impose unnecessary stress on the muscle. Stretching increases extensibility and reduces the resistance of the muscles. It also produces more efficient muscle contractions and reduces the chances of injury or soreness. In addition, an integral part of cooling down is static stretching of the muscles that have been used during exercise. The stretching will increase the exit of lactic acid from the muscles, prevent blood pooling in the muscles, and reduce muscle soreness.

18. Why is it important to utilize the full range of motion when performing strengthening exercises?

BALLISTIC STRETCHING

Ballistic stretching, on the other hand, involves rapid bouncing, jerking movements, which have the potential for injuring soft muscle and joint tissue. The ballistic method of jerking and bouncing actually invokes what is called a stretch reflex, wherein the muscle senses that it is overextended and contracts as a means of protection. The purpose of stretching is to lengthen the muscle, not shorten it; therefore, ballistic stretching is counterproductive.

PROPRIOCEPTIVE NEUROMUSCULAR FACILITATION (PNF)

An alternative method of stretching is to precede a static stretch with an isometric contraction of the muscle group to be stretched. This stretching method is called **proprioceptive neuromuscular facilitation (PNF).** This method is effective in improving muscle relaxation and leads to increased flexibility. The procedure generally requires two people. A partner moves the limb passively through its range of motion. After reaching the end point of the range of motion, the muscle is isometrically contracted for six to ten seconds against the partner's resistance; the muscle then relaxes and is again stretched using static techniques. This method is also called contract-relax (c-R). It is vital that the partner is adequately trained in the technique so that injury will not result.

It is essential in sports activities that an extremity be capable of moving through a nonrestricted range of motion. All three methods of stretching have been shown to improve flexibility. Ballistic stretching is seldom utilized because of the increased chance of injury or soreness, even though many of our activities are ballistic in nature. Static stretching is the most widely utilized because it is easy to perform, safe, and does not require a partner. PNF stretching techniques have been shown to produce dramatic increases in range of motion in a very short time. The main disadvantage with PNF stretching is that it requires a trained partner.

STRETCHING AND WARM-UP PRINCIPLES

1. No matter what the nature of the exercise to come, a slow, gradual warm-up consisting of calisthenics, stretching, and slow jogging, should always precede exercise, even if you are highly trained.
2. Be ready to make minor adjustments to your stretching routine. You may be more flexible on some days than others.
3. Your warm-up should last ten to fifteen minutes.
4. Stretching following mild jogging should be slow but thorough.

5. Initial stretching should be gentle and specific to the muscles that will recieve the most stress.
6. The muscle must be stretched beyond its normal range, but not to the point of pain.
7. Stretch only to the point you feel tightness and resistance.
8. Avoid overstretching the ligaments and joint capsule.
9. Take caution with stretching exercises of the neck and lower back.
10. Always stretch slowly and in control.
11. Don't hold your breath while stretching.
12. Stretch at least three times a week for maximum results.
13. When utilizing PNF, make sure your partner is well trained in the technique.
14. Jogging should be conducted at an intensity and rate specific to your anticipated activity and level of fitness.
15. Only a few minutes should lapse between the completion of the warm-up and the activity.
16. Experiment with different types of warm-ups. Find the one that best fits your body. The warm-up should feel good.
17. A portion of the warm-up exercise should consist of skill drills and other skilled movements related to the anticipated activity to follow the warm-up.
18. Remember to stretch and cool down following the activity.

Figures 13.1 through 13.18 show a comprehensive group of stretching exercises that include the most commonly utilized muscles in the body and those that generally experience the most stress.

Figure 13.1 BEHIND THE NECK SHOULDER STRETCH. FROM A STANDING POSITION, FLEX RIGHT ARM AND RAISE ELBOW ABOVE HEAD. RIGHT HAND PALM DOWN BEHIND BACK. PLACE LEFT ARM, ELBOW FLEXED, BEHIND BACK AND BRING FINGERS TOGETHER. YOU MAY USE A STICK IF YOU CANNOT CONNECT FINGERS. REPEAT WITH LEFT ARM. HOLD FOR FIFTEEN SECONDS AND REPEAT FIVE TIMES.

Muscles Stretched:

Internal/External Rotators

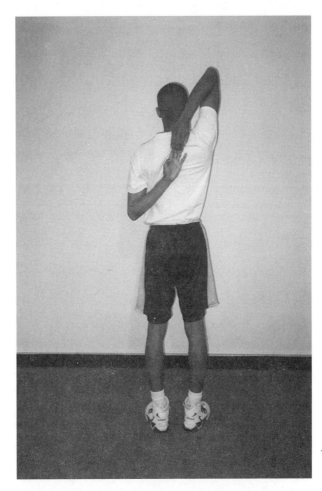

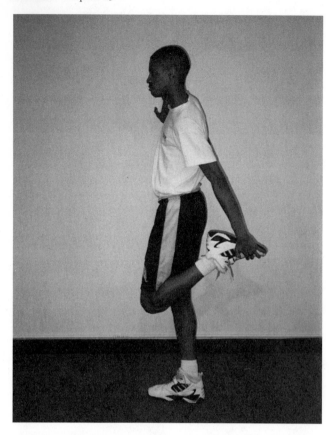

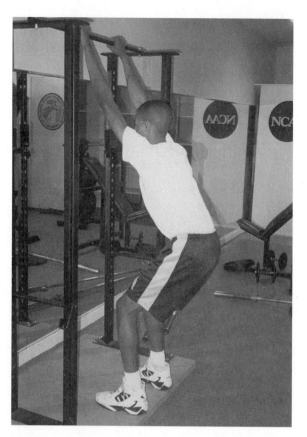

Figure 13.2 FRONT-LEG STRETCH. LEAN AGAINST A WALL. BRING YOUR LEFT FOOT UP BEHIND YOU. GRASP THE FOOT WITH YOUR LEFT HAND. HOLD FOR FIFTEEN SECONDS. REPEAT FIVE TIMES FOR EACH LEG. CAUTION: DO NOT PULL TOWARD BUTTOCKS. ONLY GRASP ANKLE.

Muscles Stretched:
Quadriceps.

Figure 13.3 SHOULDER AND ARM STRETCH. PLACE BOTH HANDS SHOULDER-WIDTH APART ON A LEDGE OR STATIONARY BAR. BEND KNEES SLIGHTLY AND LET UPPER BODY DROP DOWN. ADJUST HEIGHT OF HANDS AND DEGREE OF KNEE BEND TO INCREASE OR DECREASE STRETCH. HOLD FOR FIFTEEN SECONDS. REPEAT FIVE TIMES.

Muscles Stretched:
Shoulder Girdle.

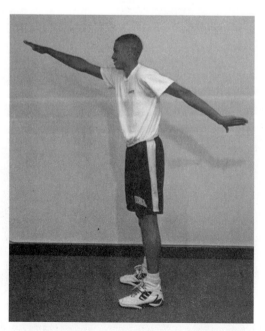

Figure 13.4 FORWARD-AND-BACK-ARM STRETCH. STAND WITH YOUR FEET SHOULDER-WIDTH APART. BEND FORWARD ABOUT TWENTY DEGREES FROM THE WAIST. EXTEND YOUR LEFT ARM TO THE FRONT AND YOUR RIGHT ARM TO THE REAR. HOLD YOUR ARMS SHOULDER HIGH FOR FIFTEEN SECONDS. REPEAT FIVE TIMES. THEN REVERSE ARM POSITIONS AND REPEAT FIVE TIMES.

Muscles Stretched:
Obliques, Back.

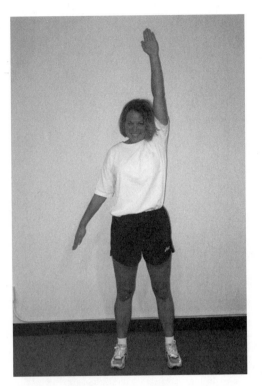

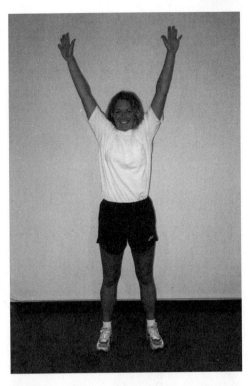

Figure 13.5 HIGH-LOW ARM STRETCH. STAND WITH YOUR FEET SHOULDER-WIDTH APART. EXTEND YOUR RIGHT ARM STRAIGHT UP FROM YOUR BODY AND EXTEND YOUR LEFT ARM STRAIGHT DOWN. HOLD THE STRETCH FOR FIFTEEN SECONDS. REPEAT FIVE TIMES. THEN REVERSE ARM POSITIONS AND REPEAT FIVE TIMES.

Muscles Stretched:
Shoulder, Chest, Obliques.

Figure 13.6 ARM AND LEG STRETCH. STAND WITH YOUR FEET SHOULDER-WIDTH APART. RAISE YOUR EXTENDED ARMS OVERHEAD. PLACE YOUR WEIGHT ON YOUR TOES AND STRETCH TO THE SKY. HOLD FOR FIFTEEN SECONDS. REPEAT FIVE TIMES.

Muscles Stretched:
Trunk, Shoulder Girdle.

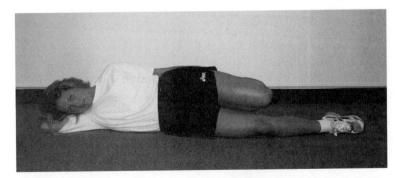

Figure 13.7 QUADRICEPS STRETCH. WHILE LYING ON YOUR RIGHT SIDE, FLEX THE KNEE OF YOUR LEFT LEG AND GRAB THE ANKLE WITH YOUR LEFT HAND. GRADUALLY MOVE YOUR HIP FORWARD UNTIL A GOOD STRETCH IS FELT ON THE THIGH. HOLD FOR FIFTEEN SECONDS. REPEAT FIVE TIMES. REPEAT FOR THE RIGHT LEG WHILE LYING ON YOUR RIGHT SIDE. CAUTION: DO NOT PULL THE ANKLE. LET THE HIP MOVEMENT CREATE THE STRETCH.

Muscles Stretched:
Quadriceps.

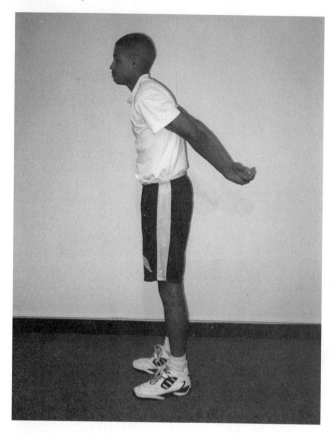

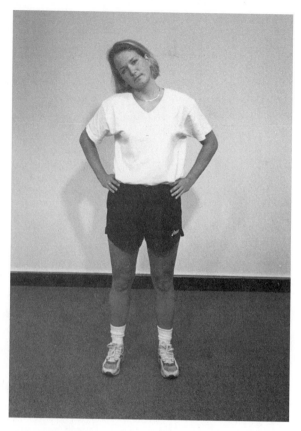

Figure 13.8 UPPER-CHEST STRETCH. STAND WITH YOUR FEET SLIGHTLY APART. GRASP YOUR HANDS BEHIND YOUR BACK AND RAISE YOUR ARMS. HOLD FOR FIFTEEN SECONDS. REPEAT FIVE TIMES.

Muscles Stretched:

Anterior Shoulder, Rotators.

Figure 13.9 NECK STRETCH. STAND WITH YOUR HANDS ON YOUR HIPS. FLEX YOUR HEAD TOWARD YOUR RIGHT SHOULDER. HOLD FOR FIFTEEN SECONDS. THEN FLEX YOUR HEAD TOWARD YOUR LEFT SHOULDER AND HOLD FOR FIFTEEN SECONDS. REPEAT FIVE TIMES.

Muscles Stretched:

Lateral Neck.

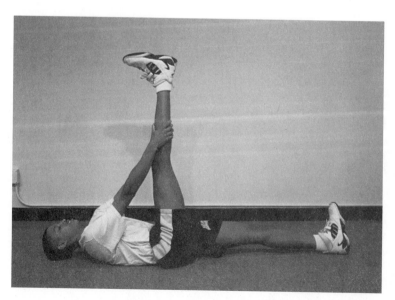

Figure 13.10

HAMSTRING STRETCH. LIE FLAT ON BACK. RAISE ONE LEG STRAIGHT UP WITH KNEE EXTENDED AND ANKLE FLEXED AT 90 DEGREES. GRASP LEG AROUND CALF AND PULL TOWARD HEAD. REPEAT WITH OPPOSITE LEG. HOLD FOR FIFTEEN SECONDS AND REPEAT THREE TIMES.

Muscles Stretched:

Hamstring.

Figure 13.11
MODIFIED HURDLER STRETCH.
SIT WITH YOUR LEFT LEG
EXTENDED AND YOUR RIGHT
LEG CROSSED IN FRONT WITH
THE HEEL NEAR YOUR
CROTCH. REACH FORWARD
WITH YOUR LEFT ARM AS FAR
AS POSSIBLE. BEND KNEE
SLIGHTLY. HOLD FOR FIFTEEN
SECONDS. REPEAT FIVE TIMES
FOR EACH LEG.

Muscles Stretched:

Hamstrings, Gastrocnemius,
Lower Back.

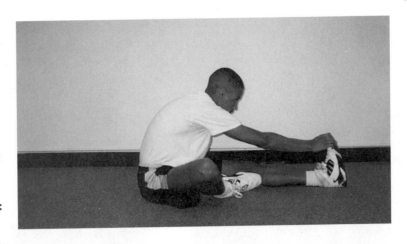

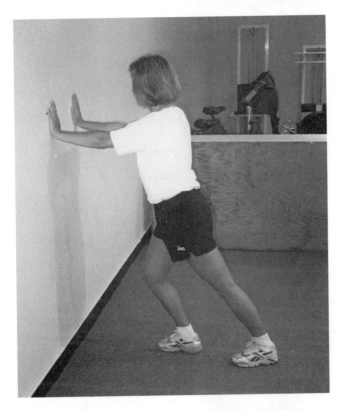

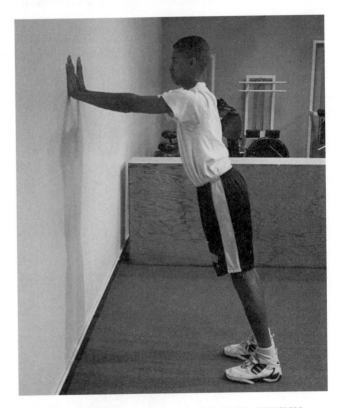

Figure 13.12 WALL LEAN AND HEEL STRETCH.
STAND ABOUT THREE FEET FROM THE WALL, WITH ONE
FOOT IN FRONT OF THE OTHER. BEND THE FRONT KNEE
SLIGHTLY, AND KEEP THE BACK LEG FULLY EXTENDED.
KEEP HEELS ON THE GROUND. HOLD FOR FIFTEEN
SECONDS. REPEAT FIVE TIMES FOR EACH LEG.

Muscles Stretched:

Hamstrings, Gastrocnemius.

Figure 13.13 LOWER-LEG AND HEEL STRETCH.
(THE ACHILLES TENDON IS A LARGE TENDON
CONNECTING THE CALF MUSCLE TO THE HEEL.) FACE A
WALL AND STAND APPROXIMATELY THREE FEET IN
FRONT OF IT WITH YOUR FEET SEVERAL INCHES APART.
PLACE YOUR OUTSTRETCHED HANDS ON THE WALL
WHILE KEEPING YOUR FEET FLAT ON THE FLOOR.
GRADUALLY LEAN FORWARD TOWARD THE WALL. HOLD
THE STRETCH FOR TEN SECONDS. REPEAT FIVE TIMES.

Muscles Stretched:

Gastrocnemius.

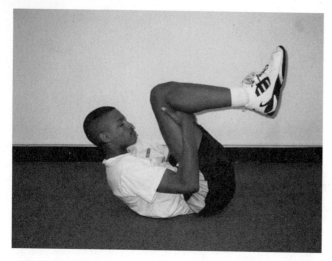

Figure 13.14 BACK STRETCH. WHILE LYING ON YOUR BACK, BRING BOTH OF YOUR KNEES TO YOUR CHEST. GRASP BOTH OF YOUR LEGS BEHIND THE KNEES AND PULL THE KNEES TOWARD YOUR CHEST. HOLD FOR TEN SECONDS. REPEAT TEN TIMES.

Muscles Stretched:

Lower Back, Gluteus, Hamstrings.

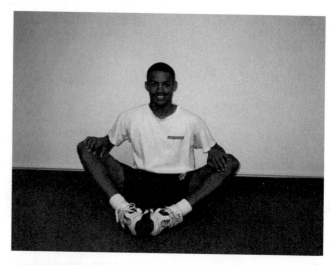

Figure 13.15 GROIN STRETCH. SIT ON THE FLOOR WITH THE SOLES OF YOUR FEET TOUCHING IN FRONT OF YOU. GRADUALLY PUSH YOUR KNEES DOWN AS FAR AS POSSIBLE. HOLD THE FINAL STRETCHED POSITION FOR TEN SECONDS. REPEAT FIVE TIMES. EACH DAY TRY TO PUSH YOUR KNEES CLOSER TO THE FLOOR.

Muscles Stretched:

Adductors.

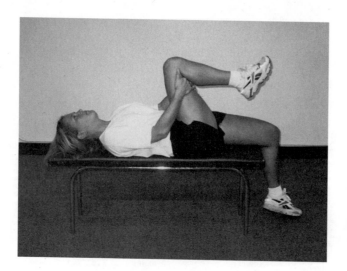

Figure 13.16 HIP FLEXOR. LIE ON YOUR BACK ON A BENCH WITH YOUR LEGS OVER THE EDGE OF THE BENCH. BRING YOUR RIGHT KNEE TO YOUR CHEST. USE BOTH OF YOUR HANDS ON YOUR KNEECAP TO GRADUALLY PRESS THE KNEE TOWARD YOUR ARMPIT. HOLD FOR FIFTEEN SECONDS. REPEAT FIVE TIMES FOR EACH LEG. CAUTION: DO NOT APPLY DOWNWARD PRESSURE WITH HAND ON KNEE JOINT.

Muscles Stretched:

Hamstrings, Gluteus.

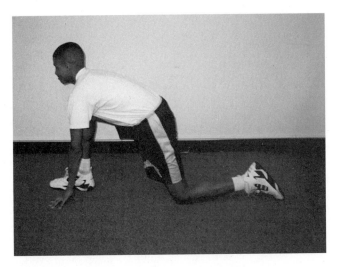

Figure 13.17 LEG AND GROIN STRETCH. MOVE ONE LEG FORWARD UNTIL THE KNEE OF THE FRONT LEG IS DIRECTLY OVER THE ANKLE. REST THE BACK KNEE ON THE FLOOR. WITHOUT CHANGING LEG POSITION, LOWER THE FRONT HIP DOWNWARD TO CREATE A STRETCH. HOLD FOR FIFTEEN SECONDS. REPEAT FIVE TIMES. CHANGE POSITION AND REPEAT FOR THE OTHER LEG.

Muscles Stretched:

Hip Flexors, Rectus Femoris, Iliopsoas.

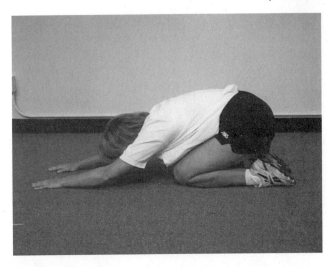

Figure 13.18 LOWER BACK AND HIP STRETCH. GET DOWN ON ALL FOURS BY PLACING YOUR HANDS AND KNEES ON THE FLOOR. LEAN BACK ONTO YOUR HEELS, EXTEND YOUR ARMS, AND PLACE YOUR CHEST ON THE FLOOR. HOLD FOR FIFTEEN SECONDS. REPEAT FIVE TIMES.

Muscles Stretched:

Lower Back, Gluteus.

Glossary

Achilles Tendon   A large tendon connecting the calf muscle to the heel.
Ballistic Stretching   Rapid bouncing, jerking types of muscle movements.
Flexibility   The range and the extent of the movement of a joint.
Hamstring   A group of three muscles in the upper leg that flex the leg at the knee.
Hyperextension   Extension beyond the normal range of the joint structure.
Proprioceptive Neuromuscular Facilitation (PNF)   A method of stretching where an isometric contraction of the muscle group to be stretched precedes a static stretch.
Static Stretching   A stretching method that consists of stretching the muscle slowly and gradually.
Warm-Up   Exercises performed immediately before physical activity to prepare the heart, lungs, and muscles to adequately meet the demands of rigorous exercise.

chapter 14

injuries

Objectives

After studying this chapter you should be able to:

1. Describe the major reasons for injury in strength training.
2. Define muscle balance and positioning.
3. Describe important safety procedures.
4. Describe common injuries, prevention, and treatment.

Many of the injuries that occur during strength training are avoidable. A number of individuals are injured because they take unnecessary risks such as trying to lift too much weight, use incorrect techniques, or ignore safety guidelines. They may be unaware of how easily they can injure themselves. An injury can force you to stop your program or cut back until you recover. The best way to insure steady progress is to avoid injury.

Weight training, because it places great stress on muscles, tendons, and ligaments, is an activity in which minor injuries may occur. Most, however, can be avoided if some simple rules are followed.

1. Lift Progressively.
   Start with a light weight and progressively add resistance with each set. Do not start with your heaviest set first, as the muscles and tendons are not prepared for such sudden exertion.
2. Insure Muscle Balance.
   You should exercise opposite muscle groups (prime mover and antagonist) in your workout to insure proper muscle balance.
3. Maintain Good Positioning.
   Proper positioning is important in maintaining the correct alignment of the skeletal system and in positioning the exercised muscles for maximum force development.
4. Lift Safely.
   Review chapter 3.
5. Always use the proper equipment.
   Review chapter 3.
6. Overtraining.
   The most common cause of injury to lifters is training error. For the beginner it is doing too much too soon, resulting in overfatiguing the muscle, with an inadequate rest and rehabilitation interval. The muscles respond fairly rapidly to the increased demand placed upon them with a lifting program. Tendons and ligaments, however, take significantly longer to adapt to the added stress and will require a more progressive adaptation period if injury is to be avoided.

The key to avoiding overtraining is to make sure you have adequate rest. The rest period is when the muscle recovers and when the gains in strength and endurance occur. You need to listen to your body and adapt the intensity and duration of your exercise program to the needs and ability of your body to recover. There will be times when the best workout you could have is a light workout or no workout at all.

One of the first signs of overtraining is mental staleness. If rest is insufficient in either quality or quantity, then often sickness such as colds or flu occurs.

A common progression is:

1. staleness or slump
2. sickness
3. injury

If you learn to listen to your body, 2 and 3 can be avoided.

COMMON INJURIES

Injuries may also result from overuse and lack of rest for the muscles and tendons. The belly of the muscle contains the contractile elements and is where the work of the muscle is performed. The tendons are tough fibers that connect the muscle to the bones.

Lifting injuries can be classified into several groups:

1. tendinitis
2. strains and sprains
3. bursitis
4. dislocations and fractures

Tendinitis

Tendinitis is an inflammation of a tendon and is characterized by swelling and tenderness. It is usually caused by a repeated irritation to an area. This injury is most common when many repetitions of a lift are performed. Common sites for tendinitis are the Achilles tendon in the back of the heel, the patella tendon of the knee, tendons in the shoulder and elbows, and also tendons in the wrist and hand.

Strains and Sprains

A strain is a tear in the muscle and/or tendon. Strains can occur when the muscle is not warmed up properly, when a twisting or jerking occurs during the lift, when significant force is applied too rapidly (such as in raising or lowering the weight too quickly), or when a previously injured muscle is returned to heavy exercise without adequate rehabilitation.

A sprain is a tear in a ligament. Ligaments are structures that hold the bones together, such as those in the knee and ankle. The same circumstances that were listed as causing strains can also cause sprains.

Strains and sprains are classified by degrees:

First degree—tearing of a few fibers, resulting in mild tenderness and slight swelling.
Second degree—partial disruption of the involved tissues, causing more tenderness and swelling.
Third degree—complete tearing of the tissue, resulting in significant pain and swelling. The joint may be difficult to move and/or the torn muscle may exhibit a bulge.

Strains and sprains are the most common types of lifting injuries and occur most often in the following areas:

Strains
1. chest and back muscles (shoulder girdle)
2. arm muscles (shoulder girdle)
3. hamstrings
4. quadriceps

19. Assume you are initiating a new recruit to the strength training room. What safety precautions will you emphasize?

Sprains
1. knee
2. wrist
3. ankle

Bursitis

Another common injury in lifters is bursitis. Bursitis is an inflammation of a bursa, which is a sac that contains fluid. This sac is strategically located in or near joints to assist in the joint or tendon movement. Sometimes the sac becomes irritated from abrasion or gets pinched during a joint movement, resulting in inflammation, tenderness, and pain. The shoulder is the most common site of bursitis for lifters, with bursitis in the knees, hips, and elbows as the next most common sites.

Dislocation and Fractures

A dislocation is a separation of the joint surface, which can be either partial or complete. The shoulder, elbow, wrist, knee, and vertebrae are the most common sites for this injury. In other sports these usually occur by trauma, such as a collision in football or a fall in gymnastics. In weight training they can occur when incorrect alignment of a body part occurs during the lift, such as twisting the neck or back while lifting. Dislocation can also occur as a result of a severe sprain or strain that occurs during the lift. Some people, because of their joint structure, are susceptible to dislocation and should exercise caution. Have spotters and insure correct body position. Dislocation usually involves significant pain and lack of mobility as well as swelling and tissue damage.

Fractures are much less common in lifting than in other sports, but they do occur. The two most common sites are the wrist and feet. The overhead lifts such as the snatch and the clean-and-press place significant stress on the wrist joint and can cause a partial crack or complete break in the bones. This causes significant swelling and pain. The other lifting related fractures occur as hairline cracks in the bones of the feet. These are sometimes referred to as fatigue fractures, as they usually result from high levels of stress without adequate rest in between periods of exercise. These fatigue fractures exhibit tenderness and swelling.

Most athletes will sustain some injuries during their careers. Fortunately, most of these will be minor and with a little knowledge and care can be self-treated. The key is to learn what injuries you can treat and which ones need medical attention. Much of this awareness is developed by listening to your body.

The following guidelines are recommended in assessing whether or not to seek medical assistance. If the following conditions exist, you should seek assistance from an athletic trainer, nurse practitioner, physical therapist, and/or a physician.

1. pain that is severe or persists
2. inability to move the injured body part
3. the injury does not appear to be healing

The following procedures should be followed immediately after an injury such as strains, sprains, and/or tendinitis or bursitis.

R. I. C. E.
- Rest
- Ice
- Compression
- Elevation

Using this regime will help relieve pain, control inflammation, and start the healing process. Let's examine each briefly.

Rest

In severe strains, sprains, bursitis, tendinitis, and in all fractures, rest is required, and prolonged rest may be essential to recovery. Your physician should be your guide.

In less severe cases, however, complete rest may not be required. Within a few days of an injury the tissues begin to repair themselves. Proper rehabilitation exercises can aid in the repair by flushing away the injury-produced by-products from the tissue and by bringing blood and nutrients to the area. Movement will help restore the functional ability of the muscle and allow for a quicker return to your sport. Allow the pain level and type of pain to be your guide. If the pain is sharp, throbbing, and/or very severe, then exercise or movement is not indicated. If, however, there is only minor pain, then movement may aid the healing process.

Ice

Ice is important because it reduces the pain and swelling by constricting blood and lymph vessels. Ice should be placed on the injured area as soon as possible after the injury. Ice should be applied for about thirty minutes on a schedule of on for five minutes, off for five minutes, on again for five minutes, and so on.

Compression

Wrapping the injured part with an elastic bandage will compress the area and limit swelling. Be careful not to wrap the part too tightly as the blood supply will be cut off. If the part becomes numb and/or turns blue, then the wrapping is too tight. The wrapping should remain on for twenty to thirty minutes, then released for fifteen minutes to insure adequate circulation. This process may be repeated.

Elevation

Elevating the body part helps drain excess fluid from the area and along with compression can help limit muscular bleeding and swelling. It may be advisable to elevate the part while sleeping.

Other Remedies

Aspirin and Ibuprofen

Aspirin is a powerful anti-inflammatory agent and can be effective in reducing swelling and relieving pain. If you experience stomach upset with aspirin, you can try buffered aspirin (such as Bufferin). Non-aspirin pain relievers that contain acetaminophen such as Tylenol can reduce pain but are not thought to diminish inflammation. Ibuprofen can be purchased over the counter under the names Advil and Pamprin.

Cortisone, Butazone

The anti-inflammatory agents cortisone and butazone are prescription drugs. They should be prescribed and administered only by a physician and are usually reserved for severe cases.

Heat

Heat such as hot baths, analgesic balm, and heating pads can be helpful in aiding healing but should not be used on an injury until swelling is eliminated or significantly reduced. The rule of thumb is ice for twenty-four to forty-eight hours and then heat if the swelling has been eliminated.

Rehabilitation

You should begin gently with range of motion exercises as soon as you can comfortably do so, unless your doctor recommends you not do so. The sooner you begin to use the muscles, the faster you will recover. Moderation is the key! Excessive pain means you are overdoing it!

If you have consulted a physician, athletic trainer, or physical therapist, ask him or her to recommend rehabilitation exercises.

Try to learn something from each injury. Some injuries are due to accidents, such as dropping a weight on your foot. In this case all you might learn is that you need to be more careful, pay better attention to detail, or refrain from lifting weights when you are not mentally involved in the activity.

For other injuries, however, you should try to determine:

1. What is the injury? (medical personnel can help you if your anatomy background is weak).
2. What caused the injury?
3. How you can avoid such an injury?

If you answer these questions, you will be better able to prevent injuries in the future.

20. Ice and heat are often used in the treatment of injuries. What are the guidelines for the application of each?

THE FAR SIDE   By GARY LARSON

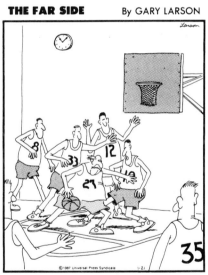

Unbeknownst to most historians, Einstein started down the road of professional basketball before an ankle injury diverted him into science.

Glossary

Bursitis   Inflammation of the bursae sac.
Dislocation   Separation of a joint surface.
Muscle Balance   Procedure where opposite muscle groups are exercised to insure proper muscle balance.
Sprain   An injury to the ligament.
Strain   An injury to the muscle or tendon.
Tendinitis   Inflammation of the tendon.

chapter 15

nutrition

Objectives

After studying this chapter you should be able to:

1. Define and describe major nutritional constituents; carbohydrates, fats, proteins, vitamins, minerals, and water.

2. Describe the energy system for muscle contraction.

3. Describe criteria for diet rating.

4. Describe weight loss and weight gain procedures.

5. Describe the Food Guide Pyramid.

NUTRITIONAL CONCEPTS

Your dietary needs for strength training or other physically active programs are not very different from those recommended for all healthy individuals. Rigorous exercise programs, however, require more energy expenditure than a sedentary lifestyle. As a result you may need to consume additional calories; the exact amount will depend on the intensity of training, your age, sex, body composition, and your present fitness level. See table 15.1 for a general estimation of your caloric needs. A diet that is deficient in the basic nutritional requirements will interfere with your strength training goals by producing early fatigue, reducing your performance level, and in some cases producing physical deterioration. On the other hand there is no evidence that taking additional dietary supplements (vitamins, protein, amino acids etc.) will increase performance levels. In fact, large doses of some supplements, such as fat-soluble vitamins, may be detrimental to your health.

NUTRITIONAL REQUIREMENTS

The major nutritional requirements are carbohydrates, protein, fats, minerals, vitamins, and water.

Carbohydrates

Carbohydrates are chemical compounds containing carbon, hydrogen, and oxygen. Examples are starches, grain products, fruits, vegetables, sugars, and milk. Carbohydrates are the most efficient fuel for the body as they are most easily broken down. They should supply fifty-five to sixty percent of daily calories for the average person and sixty to eighty percent for endurance athletes. No more than ten percent of your total calories should come from simple carbohydrates (sugars). The remaining carbohydrates should be complex carbohydrates (starch). Carbohydrates can increase energy reserves (glycogen) in muscles and liver, thus prolonging the time before exhaustion during vigorous exercise.

Proteins

The main function of protein is the building and repair of tissue. It is an energy source only when fats and carbohydrates are not available. Excellent sources of protein are eggs, meat, fish, poultry, dried beans, peas, nuts, milk, and cheese. Protein needs of sedentary and most active people are about the same. The adult requirements are approximately twelve percent of total calories. The Food and Nutrition Board recommends

Table 15.1

Daily Caloric Needs (Determined by Multiplying Body Weight in Pounds with the Appropriate Number Relating to Activity Level).		
Physical Activity	**Women**	**Men**
Sedentary	14	16
Moderately active	18	21
Active	22	26

0.8 grams of protein per kilogram of body weight. Protein supplements are unnecessary and expensive. Excess protein will not build muscles, only exercise will. Extra protein is broken down and stored as fat.

Fats

Fats belong to a class of compounds called lipids and supply energy and promote absorption of fat-soluble vitamins. They provide the primary fuel for prolonged endurance type exercise. Less than thirty percent of your daily calories should come from fat and less than ten percent from saturated fat. Avoid fatty foods before exercise as they require three to four hours to digest. Do not confuse body fat and dietary fat. Body fat is the stored form of excess caloric intake in either protein, carbohydrate, or fat.

Vitamins

Vitamins' main function is the metabolism of carbohydrates, proteins, and fats to produce energy. These organic compounds are needed in only small amounts by the body.

Individuals involved in vigorous physical activity do not require supplementary vitamins. If your caloric intake comes from a varied balanced diet high in complex carbohydrates, it should provide all the vitamins you need. Contrary to popular belief, vitamins do not provide energy or build muscle. There is no evidence of any vitamin improving physical performance. See appendix G for vitamin table.

Minerals

Minerals regulate body processes, maintain body tissue, and aid in metabolism. A varied diet generally provides enough minerals for active people, with the possible exception of iron for women. Women should also consume at least 1000 milligrams of calcium per day to protect against the onset of osteoporosis. Losses of sodium and potassium through perspiration are minimal during exercise and are usually replenished by a normal diet. Salt tablets are not necessary and may be detrimental. Table 15.2 shows current and recommended nutritional allowances, as well as nutritional allowances recommended for the high-energy needs of vigorous physical exercise. See appendix G for mineral table.

WATER

Water is the most essential nutrient. One can exist for weeks without proteins, fats, vitamins, and minerals. Without water, however, one would perish in a few days. It is vital in the body because it dissolves substances, lubricates structures such as joints, and provides a way to transport nutrients and waste. Our body cells are mostly composed of water, which makes up approximately sixty percent of our total weight. In

21. What is the most important element in your diet? How much of it should you consume each day, and how long can you do without any of it?

Table 15.2

	Current	Recommended by American Heart Association	Recommended for High-Energy Needs
Current, Recommended, and High-Energy Nutritional Allowances			
Fats	42%	30%	10 to 20%
Protein	12%	12%	10 to 12%
Complex carbohydrates	22%	48%	60 to 80%
Sugar	24%	10%	5 to 10%

extremely hot weather, the body's ability to conserve water can be negatively affected. Water is a critical element for a physically active person in these circumstances. The bulk of our dietary needs comes from water (about 10 cups a day from a combination of foods, fluids, and water itself).

ENERGY FOR MUSCLE CONTRACTION

The basic energy sources for muscles, ATP (adenosine triphosphate) and PC (phosphocreatine), are produced by the body. A muscle will expend its entire store of these compounds in only a few seconds of exercise. Depending on the type and duration of exercise, the ATP in the muscles is resupplied either by carbohydrates (glucose in blood or glycogen in the muscle or liver) or stored fats. The duration and intensity of exercise will determine what type of fuel the muscle will use for energy. Exercises lasting one to two minutes are fueled by the anaerobic process (without oxygen) since little oxygen is available during this period of time. Sprinting, weight lifting, and jumping are examples of anaerobic activities. If the exercise continues past two minutes, the body is required to draw upon oxygen (aerobic). The oxygen system can utilize both glycogen and fats for fuel for the production of ATP. Activities that are low to moderate in intensity and of long duration, such as jogging, long-distance swimming, and cross-country skiing, use fat as their primary energy source.

DIETS

The world is full of various diets. However, no matter which diets are used (except for a specific medical problem), each diet should be judged by the following criteria:

Diet Rating

1. Does the diet provide a reasonable number of kcalories (kcal), enough to maintain weight but not an excess; and if a reduction diet, not fewer than 1200 kcal for the average-size person?
2. Does it provide enough, but not too much, protein, at least the recommended intake or RDA (Recommended Daily Allowance), but not more than twice as much?
3. Does it provide enough fat for satiety, but not so much fat as to exceed current recommendations, between twenty and thirty-five percent of the kcal from fat?

Table 15.3

How to Identify a Fraud

1. The use of anecdotes and testimonials to support claims.
2. Promises of quick, dramatic increases in strength and endurance.
3. Promotional literature devoid of reliable scientific research.
4. The claim that natural vitamins are better than synthetic ones.
5. The citing of so-called experts who may well be inexperienced and unknowledgeable.
6. An indication that their claims are suppressed by the medical community because they are controversial.
7. The advice that taking vitamin supplements will give you energy.
8. Literature suggests that people should take vitamin and mineral supplements just to be on the safe side.
9. The use of words like "natural" and "organic."
10. Warnings that you cannot get enough nutrients from your diet no matter how hard you try.

4. Does it provide enough carbohydrates to spare protein and prevent ketosis, 100 grams of carbohydrate for the average-size person? Is it mostly complex carbohydrate, not more than twenty percent of the kcal as concentrated sugar?
5. Does it offer a balanced assortment of vitamins and minerals from whole food sources in all four food groups (milk and milk products; meat, fish, poultry, and eggs; legumes, fruits, and vegetables; and grains)?
6. Does it offer variety, in that different foods can be selected each day?
7. Does it consist of ordinary foods that are available locally and at prices people normally pay?

Fraudulent Claims

We are continually bombarded by unsound and unsubstantiated claims for various supplements and diet combinations that purport to increase muscle strength and endurance and boost energy. Slick advertising, along with personal and anecdotal evidence, persuade millions of individuals to use substances that are completely useless and in some cases physically harmful. Doses of dietary supplements exceeding minimum requirements have not been found to increase work performance. Most dietary claims are unfounded and not based on scientific evidence. Many of the so-called supplements commonly promoted and used have never been tested for efficacy or safety. Table 15.3 will give you some tips on how to spot the fraudulent.

If you follow the recommendations in figure 15.1, the Food Guide Pyramid, you will be on a sound basis for insuring that you are receiving a proper, nutritional diet.

"Super-Protein" Diets

Some athletes ingest large amounts of protein supplements, believing that doing so will help them build up their muscles and energy level, even though there is no scientific justification for the use of these supplements. Athletes generally do not need additional protein but additional calories in the form of complex carbohydrates to provide energy for muscle activity. Most athletes already consume twice as much protein as they can possibly use and probably are wasting about half as much as they eat.

Figure 15.1 FOOD GUIDE PYRAMID: A GUIDE TO DAILY FOOD CHOICES.

Source: FDA Consumer, June 1993.

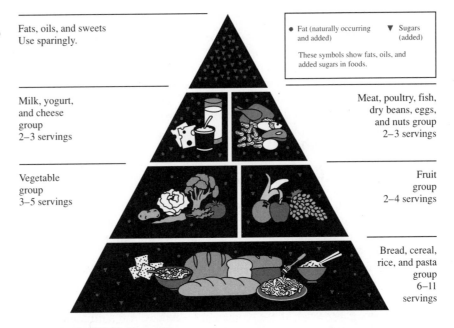

Fats, oils, and sweets
Use sparingly.

● Fat (naturally occurring and added)   ▼ Sugars (added)

These symbols show fats, oils, and added sugars in foods.

Milk, yogurt, and cheese group
2–3 servings

Meat, poultry, fish, dry beans, eggs, and nuts group
2–3 servings

Vegetable group
3–5 servings

Fruit group
2–4 servings

Bread, cereal, rice, and pasta group
6–11 servings

What is the Food Guide Pyramid?

The Pyramid is an outline of what to eat each day. It's not a rigid prescription but a general guide that lets you choose a healthful diet that's right for you.

The Pyramid calls for eating a variety of foods to get the nutrients you need and at the same time the right amount of calories to maintain a healthy weight.

The Pyramid also focuses on fat because most American diets are too high in fat, especially saturated fat.

Fat

● In general, foods that come from animals (milk and meat groups) are naturally higher in fat than foods that come from plants. But there are many low-fat dairy and lean meat choices available, and these foods can be prepared in ways that lower fat.

Fruits, vegetables, and grain products are naturally low in fat. But many popular items are prepared with fat, such as french-fried potatoes or croissants, making them higher-fat choices.

Added sugars

▼ These symbols represent sugars added to foods in processing or at the table, not the sugars found naturally in fruits and milk. It's the added sugars that provide calories with few vitamins and minerals.

Most of the added sugars in the typical American diet come from foods in the Pyramid tip—soft drinks, candy, jams, jellies, syrups, and table sugar we add to foods such as coffee or cereal.

Added sugars in the food groups come from foods such as ice cream, sweetened yogurt, chocolate milk, canned or frozen fruit with heavy syrup, and sweetened bakery products such as cakes and cookies.

What counts as a serving?

Milk, yogurt, and cheese group (2–3 servings)	Meat, poultry, fish, dry beans, eggs, and nuts group (2–3 servings)	Vegetable group (3–5 servings)	Fruit group (2–4 servings)	Bread, cereal, rice, and pasta group (6–11 servings)
1 c. milk or yogurt 1 1/2 oz. natural cheese 2 oz. processed cheese 1 c. frozen yogurt 1 1/2 c. ice cream 2 c. cottage cheese	2–3 oz. cooked, lean meat, poultry, or fish 1/3 c. nuts (Count 1/2 c. cooked dry beans, 1 egg, or 2 Tbls. peanut butter as 1 oz. meat.)	1 c. raw leafy greens 1/2 c. other kinds of vegetables (raw or cooked) 3/4 c. vegetable juice	1 medium apple, banana, orange 1/2 c. chopped, cooked, canned fruit 3/4 c. juice	1 slice bread 1/2 bun or bagel 1 oz. dry cereal 1/2 c. cooked cereal, rice, or pasta 3–4 small, plain crackers

Source: Adapted from E. N. Whitney, M. A. Boyle, *Understanding Nutrition,* 4th edition, West Publishing Co., St. Paul, MN, 1987.

It is impossible to force extra amounts of protein into the muscles just by eating more. For muscle cells to accept additional protein, additional demands have to be made upon the muscles. To make a muscle grow, you have to overload it. The muscle generally responds by taking in more nutrients and subsequently accelerating its growth.

The so-called "super-protein" diets are unnecessary, expensive, and in some cases harmful. For example, with large amounts of protein, the blood level of uric acid may increase and damage the kidneys and make the joints more susceptible to injuries. As for energy derived from protein, you burn up as much protein reading a book as running track at top speed. The body burns protein for energy only in starvation.

Vitamin and Mineral Supplemented Diets

Supplementing your diet with vitamins and minerals above the minimum daily requirement does not improve physical performance. In fact, excessive intake of vitamins A, D, and K can cause toxic effects. Minimum daily vitamin and mineral requirements are met easily through a normal, well-balanced diet.

The only exception to this may be the iron requirement of females engaged in rigorous physical activity, particularly after menstrual blood loss. These women have been found to have significantly decreased levels of iron in their blood. Since overdoses of iron can be toxic, however, these women should take iron supplements only after consulting with a physician.

Fad Diets

A number of fad diets with varying combinations of nutrients unfortunately have found wide acceptance because of media misinformation and public ignorance. Be very wary of these diets because they may have a number of dangerous consequences. For example, individuals on diets that do not allow for protein or that are low in protein may suffer a loss of muscle tissue and severe weakness. A high-fat diet, sometimes advocated in combination with high protein and very little carbohydrates, may produce a loss of nutrients and electrolytes, very high cholesterol levels, and diarrhea. A high-protein and high-fat diet with low carbohydrates may produce kidney problems, dizziness, weakness, dehydration, irritability, and uric acid formation. Low-fat diets may lead to dry skin, constipation, irritability, stiff joints, and a number of other problems.

Other fad diets that have enjoyed unwarranted popularity include the low-carbohydrate diet, "super-protein" diets, and vitamin and mineral supplemental diets. "Diet foods" and using drugs to lose weight also are discussed in this section.

22. "Super-protein" diets are advocated by some nutrition faddists. Can you name two health problems associated with the diet and explain why they occur?

BASIC NUTRITIONAL RECOMMENDATIONS

1. Increase consumption of fruits and vegetables.
2. Decrease consumption of red and organ meats and increase consumption of poultry and fish. Remember, shrimp and lobster are higher in cholesterol than other fish.
3. Decrease consumption of foods high in fat and substitute polyunsaturated and monosaturated fat for saturated fat. Reduce saturated fat consumption to about ten percent of total energy intake.
4. Substitute skim milk (nonfat milk) for whole milk.
5. Decrease consumption of butterfat, eggs, and other sources high in cholesterol. Reduce cholesterol intake to 300 milligrams a day (equivalent of one egg).
6. Decrease consumption of refined foods (cane and beet sugar) and processed foods (corn sugar, syrups, molasses, honey) that are high in sugar content.
7. Increase consumption of complex carbohydrates: grains, breads, cereals, potatoes, corn, and rice.
8. Decrease consumption of salt and foods with a high salt content.

How to Gain Weight

The best way to gain weight is to build muscle mass through careful and consistent physical training. Eat a well-balanced and nutritious diet with enough calories in the form of complex carbohydrates to support a weight gain.

How to Lose Weight

Exercise is an integral part of any weight-loss program. Approximately 3500 kcalories are contained in one pound of stored fat. If, for example, your food intake for one day is equivalent to 2200 kcalories and you burn up 2200 kcalories in your daily activity, you will be in caloric balance; you will not gain or lose weight. However, if you burn up an additional 100 kcalories a day through a vigorous exercise program, bringing your total daily expenditure to 2300 and at the same time still taking in only 2200 kcalories, you will incur a deficit of 100 kcalories a day. If you were to continue this regimen for thirty-five days you would accumulate a total caloric deficit of 3500 kcalories, which should be equal to a loss of one pound of fat. A deficit of 200 kcalories a day would result in a loss of one pound of fat in one half that time. Maximum weight loss should not exceed two pounds a week or a deficit of 1000 kcalories per day.

Glossary

Adenosine Triphosphate (ATP)   An energy-rich chemical compound stored in muscle cells; a source of immediate energy.

Carbohydrates   Chemical compounds containing carbon, hydrogen, and oxygen; examples are sugars and starches, major sources of energy.

Fats   Food stuffs containing glycerol and fatty acids.

Ketosis   The development of ketone bodies and acidosis (disruption of the acid/base balance) due to improper breakdown of fats.

Kilocalories   The amount of energy required to raise one kilogram of water one degree centigrade.

Minerals   Inorganic compounds, some of which are nutrients vital to body function. Examples include phosphorus, calcium, potassium, sodium, iron, and iodine.

Phosphocreatine   A chemical that can donate its phosphate to form ATP in the muscle.

Protein   Organic material that regulates body processes and builds and repairs body tissue.

Vitamins   Organic compounds that regulate a number of body processes and that are used in the metabolism of carbohydrates.

chapter 16

d r u g s

Objectives

After studying this chapter you should be able to:

1. Describe the present state of drug use in strength training programs.
2. Describe anabolic steroids and their physiological effect on the body.
3. Describe the American College of Sports Medicine position statement on anabolic-androgenic steroids in sport.
4. Describe the effects of amphetamines.
5. Describe the effects of growth hormones.
6. Describe the effects of cocaine.
7. Describe the effects of caffeine.

The use of drugs by professional and amateur athletes to improve performance is prevalent at all competitive levels. Athletes have always looked for that "extra edge" that will give them the advantage over their opponent. With only hundredths of seconds, or a few inches, separating the winner from the also-ran, it is not surprising that drugs, thought to increase performance, find wide acceptance. Both male and female competitive athletes are presently using a wide range of pharmacological agents in the belief that it will increase their strength, endurance, speed, power, and skill. One of the most unfortunate aspects of the use of drugs is that many athletes appear to be willing to court major health risks in order to be competitive. They believe they must resort to the use of drugs.

ANABOLIC STEROIDS

Anabolic steroids are synthetic hormones and close relatives of testosterone, the male hormone. This hormone has had its chemical structure altered so that the androgenic or masculinizing effect has been reduced and its anabolic protein producing characteristics enhanced in order to promote muscle growth. There is also speculation that small residual androgenic effects increase performance by making the athletes more aggressive and competitive, resulting in an increased intensity of training motivation. Steroids have been used frequently in medical practice for malnutrition, infection, skeletal disorders, some cancers, and growth problems. Anabolic steroids promote anabolism (muscle growth) by increasing nitrogen retention. They may convert a mildly negative nitrogen balance to a positive one, depending on adequate protein and caloric intake. They may build lean body mass and increase strength in individuals who are intensively training in heavy resistance (weight lifting) activities. They do not directly improve performance in aerobic activities such as long-distance running, skiing, or swimming.

The real possibility of harmful side effects greatly outweighs the questionable increases in performance. Table 16.1 outlines the possible side effects of anabolic steroid use in males and females.

Anabolic-androgenic steroids have been associated with adverse effects on the liver, cardiovascular system, reproductive function, and psychological status. Steroids that are alkalated at the 17-carbon position (most all oral forms) are especially dangerous because of the strong link between this chemical structure and liver dysfunction. There are also additional side effects in women and children. Some are irreversible.

The use of anabolic steroids in adolescents may result in accelerated pubescence, precocious display of secondary sexual characteristics, and possible premature closure of the ends of the long bones, thus terminating bone growth. Injectable anabolic

Table 16.1

Side Effects That Have Been Observed in Those Using Anabolic Steroids

Males

Liver damage

Impaired thyroid and pituitary function

Impaired cardiovascular function

Increased blood pressure

Prostate gland disorders

Acne, skin rash

Atrophied testes

Increased aggressiveness

Changes in libido

Gastro intestinal changes

Increased muscle cramps and spasms

Gynecomastia—development of breast-like tissue

Headaches, dizziness, nose bleeds

Females—These effects are in addition to those observed in males.

Deepening voice

Increase in facial/body hair

Acne

Clitoral enlargement

Menstrual irregulation

Increased fibrous (collagen) content of body

steroids are more potent than oral types because they do not require modification to protect from immediate metabolism by the liver. The increase in fat-free mass and possible reduction in fat mass may last for several months after the cessation of use. This fact is support for year-round random drug testing (Forbes et al. 1992). Although many claims are made for increases in performance and there is mounting anecdotal evidence, no studies have addressed whether or not steroids help or actually hinder performance. Another alarming aspect of anabolic steroid use by athletes is the potentially hazardous effect of increased aggressiveness (Pope and Katez 1988).

The American College of Sports Medicine Position Statement on Anabolic-Androgenic Steroids in Sports

It is the position of the American College of Sports Medicine that:

1. Anabolic-androgenic steroids in the presence of an adequate diet can contribute to increases in body weight, often in the lean mass compartment.
2. The gains in muscular strength achieved through high-intensity exercise and proper diet can occur by the increased use of anabolic-androgenic steroids in some individuals.
3. Anabolic-androgenic steroids do not increase aerobic power or capacity for muscular exercise.

4. Anabolic-androgenic steroids have been associated with adverse effects on the liver, cardiovascular system, and psychologic status in therapeutic trials and in limited research on athletes. Until further research is completed, the potential hazards of the use of the anabolic-androgenic steroids in athletes must include those found in therapeutic trials.

5. The use of anabolic-androgenic steroids by athletes is contrary to the rules and ethical principles of athletic competition as set forth by many of the sports governing bodies. The American College of Sports Medicine supports these ethical principles and deplores the use of anabolic-androgenic steroids by athletes.

AMPHETAMINES

Amphetamines are a group of drugs that stimulate the central nervous system of the body. They generally cause a rise in blood pressure, cardiac output, blood sugar, breathing rate, and metabolism. Athletes take amphetamines in hopes that the increased arousal level and depression of the sensation of muscle fatigue will enable them to maintain higher performance levels for longer periods of time. There is very little scientific evidence that amphetamines improve speed, performance, or increase endurance. Most of the studies report that the drugs have very little effect. Some athletes use amphetamines to "get them up" for competition or psychologically ready to compete. This practice may require the athlete to resort to the use of barbiturates to enable them to come down from the amphetamine high in order to sleep. The result is a dangerous stimulant to depressant combination. One of the dangers of taking amphetamines during exercise is that the individual may overstress the body with possible damage to the heart. Other major risks are psychological dependence and the possibility of circulatory collapse.

CAFFEINE

There is some recent evidence that caffeine may in some circumstances increase endurance in moderately strenuous activity. Caffeine facilitates the use of fat as a fuel, and increases the permeability of the muscle cell to calcium, resulting in a more efficient contraction and the sparing of glycogen in the muscles. Caffeine may also have a psychostimulating effect, causing the athlete to feel that the exercise was easier. The adverse effects of using caffeine are that some individuals encounter an allergic response, cardiac arhythmias, headaches, insomnia, irritability, and a diuretic effect.

GROWTH HORMONES

There is a major concern that growth hormones (somatotrophic hormone) will replace anabolic steroids as the new high-tech drug. Growth hormone is produced by the pituitary gland in the brain. One of its functions is to stimulate and control the tissue building process of normal growth and development. It is used medically to treat children with retarded growth syndrome. With the advancement of bioengineering it will soon be possible to synthetically produce large amounts of this hormone inexpensively. Athletes are attracted to the drug because it increases protein synthesis and fat breakdown and decreases the amount of carbohydrates used by the body. However, its use in adults can lead to symptoms similar to those of acromegaly: enlarged bones of the face, hands, and feet, overgrowth of soft tissue, and a most dangerous abnormal enlargement of cardiac tissue. This hormone is most difficult to detect in screening tests because it occurs naturally in the body.

COCAINE

Cocaine is a central nervous system stimulant that produces similar effects to caffeine. Cocaine enhances alertness and masks fatigue. It produces a state of excitement and restlessness. Euphoria, heightened self-confidence, temporary relief of depression, and suppressed appetite all result from cocaine use. As these effects wear off, the user experiences a period of depression, confusion, and dizziness. Small doses slow the heart, but larger amounts stimulate the heart. Blood pressure increases as a result of constricted blood vessels, and respiration becomes shallow and rapid. Repeated use of large doses leads to weight loss, insomnia, anxiety, and paranoid delusion. Inhaling and snorting may also result in ulceration of the nasal tissue. Death may occur due to respiratory or cardiac failure.

23. If you are asked by an athlete about the use of drugs to enhance performance, what advice and substantition for your advice will you give?

ERYTHROPOIETIN

Erythropoietin has been used as an agent to stimulate increased numbers of red cells. This substance is normally secreted by the kidneys to maintain normal red cell count. The use of erythropoietin can be extremely hazardous, leading to blood clots and infection.

BETA-ADRENERGIC AGONIST

These substances have been used in an attempt to desensitize nerve receptors to fatigue. They may cause increases in heart rate and other cardiac complications.

CARNITINE

Carnitine is produced in body cells and plays a part in activating fatty acids for energy. Supplements are not necessary.

STEROID REPLACERS

There is no evidence that steroid replacers stimulate physiological functions in the muscles similar to those of anabolic steroids. The body lacks enzymes to synthesize them (diosgenin, smilogenin). Desiccated organs also have no physiological effect. Boran, which has been commonly promoted as an increaser of testosterone, actually decreases testosterone. -1- carnitine has been promoted as a substance that increases utilization of fat, but actually it has no effect at all on fat metabolism and may result in neuromuscular problems.

CHROMIUM AND VANADIUM

Chromium and Vanadium both are proported to enhance glucose utilization; however they have no significant effect. Vanadium has been found to be effective only on diabetic rats.

Glossary

Amphetamines   Group of drugs that stimulate the central nervous system.
Anabolic Steroids   Synthetic hormone similar to male hormone testosterone that stimulates increases in muscle mass.
Anabolism   Constructive metabolism.
Androgenic   A substance that stimulates male characteristics.
Caffeine   Chemical found in coffee and tea that acts as a stimulant on the central nervous system.
Cocaine   Central nervous system stimulant derived from coca leaves.
Diuretic   A substance that increases kidney function, secretion of urine, and water loss.

References

Forbes, G. B., C. R. Porta, B. E. Haerr, and R. C. Briggs. 1992. Sequence of changes in body composition induced by testosterone and reversal of changes after drug is stopped. *Journal of American Medical Association* 2676:397–99.

Pope, H. J., and D. L. Katz. 1988. Effective and psychotic symptoms associated with anabolic steroid use. *American Journal of Psychiatry* 145:487–90.

chapter 17

equipment

Objectives

After studying this chapter you should be able to:

1. Describe the use of free weights and barbells in strength training programs.

2. Describe Cybex Knee Extension, Mini-Gym, Biodex, Cybex 600, Kin-Com 500H, Kin-Com 125E, Lido, Merac, Universal Machine, Nautilus, CAM II, Hydra Fitness, Polaris, free weights, power exercise equipment, and cardiorespiratory equipment.

EQUIPMENT

The following are the major categories of resistive exercise equipment used to train muscles:

1. Free weights and barbells. This equipment cannot control speed or resistance through the full range of movement yet produces different levels of muscle stress at different points in the range of movement. There is a place in the range of movement, the sticking point, at which the mechanical factors are least favorable and the greatest amount of muscle force is required. In very heavy loads (1 RM) the exercise produces maximum stress at only one point in the range of movement. The advantage is that this type of equipment most closely mimics the action found in ballistic sport skills such as kicking and throwing.

2. Equipment that provides controlled or constant speed and variable resistance (true isokinetic equipment controls speed). This type of equipment, including categories 3 and 4, closely mimics sport skills that require tension movements through the range of movement, such as swimming and cycling.

3. Equipment that controls a constant and variable resistance by means of a hydraulic device.

4. Equipment where speed is variable and resistance is constant (some CAM devices and concentric-eccentric devices).

5. There is currently no machine whereby muscles contract under conditions of true constant speed and true constant resistance.

RESISTANCE MACHINES

There is no question that the unique design and rapid development of resistance machines has revolutionized resistance training. Thousands of individuals, in particular women, who would not go near free weights in the past, have been attracted to resistance programs as a result of the attractiveness, comfort, novelty, and challenge provided by resistance machines.

Most resistance machines provide a forced or guided two-dimensional movement pattern for the exercise. This results in limited variation of the resistance movement because of differences in individual body size. Also, most machines support the user, resulting in reduced demands for stability and balance of the user and the load. In particular, isokinetic machines allow the muscle to be exercised to its maximum potential throughout the joint's entire range of motion. They also prove a safer alternative during rehabilitation because the resistance mechanism essentially disengages when pain or discomfort is felt. Other machines allow rehabilitation when the use of the whole body is prohibited because of weakness or injury.

STRENGTH AND MUSCLE ENDURANCE EQUIPMENT

Isokinetic Machines

Cybex Knee Extension

These are extension test machines that use electric servo-breaking to provide nearly complete accommodating resistance so that muscles shorten at a constant speed and can be maximally loaded throughout the full range of motion. They are used mainly in strength testing, rehabilitation, and research.

Mini-Gym

As a greater muscle force is applied, greater frictional forces are produced, resulting in a proportional increase in resistance and a steady movement speed. Eccentric contractions, however, cannot be performed with this equipment.

Biodex

Isokinetic, concentric and eccentric, isotonic, isometric, passive.

Cybex 600

Isokinetic, powered eccentric and concentric, continuous passive motion.

Kin-Com 500H

Isokinetic, concentric and eccentric, isotonic-concentric and eccentric, isometric, passive.

Kin-Com 125E

Isokinetic, concentric and eccentric, isotonic, concentric and eccentric, isometric, passive.

Lido

Isokinetic, concentric and eccentric, continuous passive motion, isometric, isotonic, concentric.

Merac

Isokinetic, concentric, isotonic, concentric, isometric, dynamic variable.

Universal Machine

This multi-station apparatus may use a sliding fulcrum to alter the resistance of weight blocks. It duplicates most free weight exercises.

Nautilus

A cam compensates for the variations in muscular force at different joint angles by changing the lever arm. As a result, the muscles exert maximal or near maximal force throughout the full range of motion in both positive and negative phases of muscle contraction.

CAM II

The apparatus uses pneumatic, or air, resistance by means of compressed air and pneumatic cylinders.

Hydra Fitness

This machine offers accommodating resistance that controls the speed of movement by restricting the speed of movement of hydraulic fluid through a hydraulic cylinder.

Polaris

With the Polaris device the weight to be moved is drawn over an oval-shaped plate. The muscles can move through a full range of movement in both positive and negative phases of muscle contraction.

Free Weights

Barbells and dumbbells allow exercise in both positive and negative phases of muscle contraction.

POWER EXERCISE EQUIPMENT

Power exercise devices are computerized and use artificial intelligence. They coach the individual through his or her workout, giving verbal encouragement and stating when an increase in resistance is needed.

As long as you follow the basic principles of strength training as explained in chapter 3, you may accomplish your goals with any type of equipment. Whatever you enjoy and find gives satisfaction, security, and confidence is appropriate.

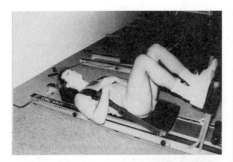
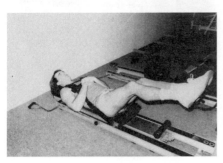
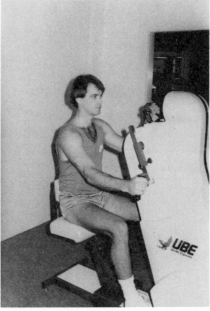
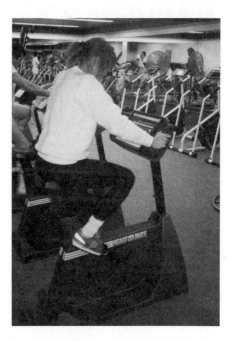

Figure 17.1 PLYOMETRIC EXERCISE FOR LOWER EXTREMITY

Figure 17.2 ARM ERGOMETER

Figure 17.3 COMPUTERIZED EXERCISE BICYCLE

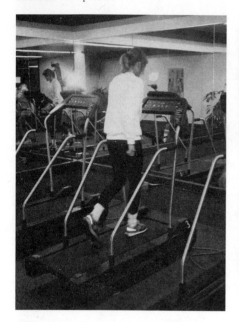

Figure 17.4 TREADMILL

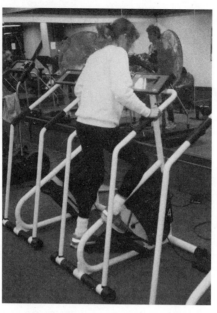

Figure 17.5 STAIR-CLIMBING MACHINE

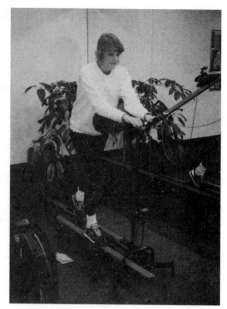

Figure 17.6 CROSS-COUNTRY SKIING MACHINE

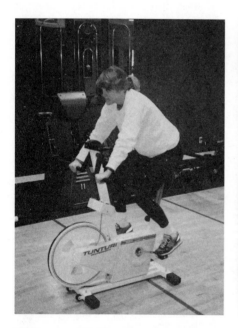

Figure 17.7 EXERCISE BICYCLE

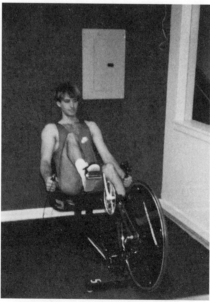

Figure 17.8 RECUMBANT EXERCISE BICYCLE

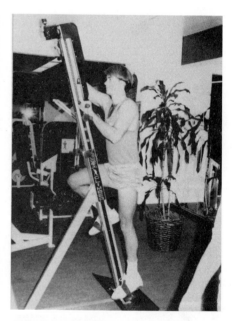

Figure 17.9 VERSA-CLIMBER

appendix a

Weight Training Activities for Various Sports

Movement	Neck flexion and extension	Shoulder shrug	Military or overhead press	Behind the neck press	Upright rowing	Bent rowing	Lat machine	Triceps extension	Lateral arm raise	Bent-arm pull-over	Biceps curl	Dumbbell curl	Bench press	Incline press	Parallel bar dip	Back hyperextension	Trunk extension	Weighted sit-ups	Hip flexion	Stiff-leg dead lift	Knee flexion	Knee extension	Squat	Hack squat	Toe raise
Baseball					×			×		×				×			×	×					×		
Basketball					×		×		×	×		×	×					×				×	×		×
Golf					×						×	×		×	×			×		×			×	×	
Gymnastics			×		×			×	×	×		×		×	×	×									
Football	×	×	×			×						×	×			×		×		×			×	×	
Soccer	×					×				×	×	×		×	×			×		×			×	×	
Rowing					×		×			×		×	×		×	×	×	×					×	×	
Tennis		×	×		×			×	×			×		×							×		×		
Wrestling	×		×			×	×	×				×	×		×	×	×	×					×	×	
Skiing		×			×			×	×			×		×	×		×	×					×	×	×
Hockey	×	×	×			×		×	×					×			×	×	×				×		
Backstroke		×		×	×			×		×				×				×					×	×	
Breaststroke						×		×	×			×		×				×			×		×		
Butterfly				×				×	×			×		×				×			×		×		
Freestyle			×		×	×		×		×		×		×	×			×	×				×		
Sprinting													×				×	×				×	×	×	×
Hurdling						×	×				×			×				×				×	×	×	×
Javelin		×	×					×		×				×				×				×	×	×	×
Long jump								×		×				×						×			×	×	
Distance running					×			×				×	×					×		×				×	×
Pole vault		×			×				×	×	×	×	×		×			×					×		
High jump										×	×		×	×				×					×	×	×
Discus and shot put			×					×			×	×	×				×	×					×	×	

Adapted from J. P. O'Shea, *Scientific Principles and Methods of Strength Fitness.* 1976. 2d. ed. McGraw-Hill Publishing Company.

appendix b

Weight Training Standards for College-Age Males

The far right column indicates the percentile ranking of each weight lifted. For example, a bench press of 125 pounds for an individual who weighs between 130 and 139 pounds would correspond to the fifty percentile. In other words, fifty percent of the individuals in the weight category pressed over 125 lbs and the remaining fifty percent pressed less than 125 lbs. The standard is based on 2,500 male college students.

Body Weight Class 120–129 lbs.

Sit-Up	Curl	Upright Rowing	Over-Head Press	Bench Press	Squat	Bent-Over Rowing	%
70	107.5	120	155	170	255	185	100
65	105	117.5	150	165	245	182.5	99.9
62.5	102.5	115	145	160	235	180	99.8
60	100	112.5	140	155	225	170	99.4
57.5	97.5	110	135	150	220	165	98.4
55	95	107.5	130	145	210	157.5	96.2
52.5	92.5	105	125	140	200	150	90.3
50	90	102.5	120	135	190	140	84.2
45	85	100	115	130	180	135	75.8
42.5	82.5	95	110	125	170	127.5	64.0
40	80	90	105	120	160	120	50.0
37.5	77.5	85	100	115	150	112.5	36.0
35	75	80	95	110	140	105	24.2
30	70	77.5	90	105	130	100	15.8
27.5	67.5	75	85	100	120	90	11.6
25	65	72.5	80	95	110	95	9.7
22.5	62.5	70	75	90	100	80	3.8
20	60	68.5	70	85	95	75	1.6
17.5	57.5	65	65	80	85	70	.2
15	55	62.5	60	75	75	65	.1
12.5	52.5	60	55	70	65	60	0

Body Weight Class 130–139 lbs.

Sit-Up	Curl	Upright Rowing	Over-Head Press	Bench Press	Squat	Bent-Over Rowing	%
70	112.5	125	165	175	265	150	100
65	110	122.5	160	170	255	145	99.9
62.5	107.5	120	155	165	245	142.5	99.8
60	105	117.5	150	160	235	140	99.4
57.5	102.5	115	145	155	230	135	98.4
55	100	112.5	140	150	220	130	96.2
52.5	97.5	110	135	145	210	125	90.3
50	95	107.5	130	140	200	120	84.2
45	90	105	125	135	190	117.5	75.8
42.5	87.5	100	120	130	180	115	64.0
40	85	95	115	125	170	110	50.0
37.5	82.5	92.5	110	120	160	105	36.0
35	80	90	105	115	150	102.5	24.2
30	75	85	100	110	140	100	15.8
27.5	72.5	80	95	105	130	95	11.6
25	70	77.5	90	100	120	90	9.7
22.5	67.5	75	85	95	110	85	3.8
20	65	72.5	80	90	105	80	1.6
17.5	60	70	75	85	95	75	.2
15	57.5	67.5	70	80	85	70	.1
12.5	55	65	65	75	80	65	0

Body Weight Class 140–149 lbs.

Sit-Up	Curl	Upright Rowing	Over-Head Press	Bench Press	Squat	Bent-Over Rowing	%
70	117.5	130	170	185	275	205	100
65	115	127.5	165	180	270	197.5	99.9
62.5	112.5	125	160	175	260	190	99.8
60	110	122.5	155	170	250	180	99.4
57.5	107.5	120	150	165	240	175	98.4
55	105	117.5	145	160	230	167.5	96.2
52.5	102.5	115	140	155	220	160	90.3
50	100	112.5	135	150	210	150	84.2
45	95	110	130	145	200	145	75.8
42.5	92.5	107.5	125	140	190	137.5	64.0
40	90	105	120	135	180	130	50.0
37.5	87.5	102.5	115	130	170	122.5	36.0
35	85	100	110	125	160	115	24.2
30	82.5	95	105	120	150	110	15.8
27.5	80	90	100	115	140	100	11.6
25	77.5	87.5	95	110	130	95	9.7
22.5	75	85	90	105	120	90	3.8
20	72.5	82.5	85	100	115	85	1.6
17.5	70	80	80	95	105	80	.2
15	67.5	77.5	75	90	100	75	.1
12.5	65	75	70	85	95	70	0

Body Weight Class 150–159 lbs.

Sit-Up	Curl	Upright Rowing	Over-Head Press	Bench Press	Squat	Bent-Over Rowing	%
75	122.5	135	175	195	290	210	100
72.5	120	132.5	170	190	285	202.5	99.9
70	117.5	130	165	185	275	195	99.8
65	115	127.5	160	180	267	185	99.4
62.5	112.5	125	155	175	255	180	98.4
60	110	122.5	150	170	245	172.5	96.2
57.5	107.5	120	145	165	235	165	90.3
55	105	117.5	140	160	225	155	84.2
50	100	115	135	155	215	150	75.8
47.5	97.5	112.5	130	150	205	142.5	64.0
45	95	110	125	145	195	135	50.0
42.5	92.5	107.5	120	140	185	127.5	36.0
40	90	105	115	135	175	120	24.2
35	85	102.5	110	130	165	115	15.8
32.5	82.5	100	105	125	155	105	11.6
30	80.5	97.5	100	120	145	100	9.7
27.5	77.5	95	92.5	115	135	95	3.8
25	75	92.5	90	110	125	90	1.6
20	72.5	90	85	105	120	85	.2
17.5	70	87.5	80	100	115	80	.1
15	67.5	85	75	95	110	75	0

Body Weight Class 160–169 lbs.

Sit-Up	Curl	Upright Rowing	Over-Head Press	Bench Press	Squat	Bent-Over Rowing	%
75	125	140	180	205	305	215	100
72.5	122.5	137.5	175	200	300	207.5	99.9
70	120	135	170	195	290	200	99.8
65	117.5	132.5	165	190	280	190	99.4
62.5	115	130	160	185	270	185	98.4
60	112.5	127.5	155	180	260	177.5	96.2
57.5	110	125	150	175	250	170	90.3
55	107.5	122.5	145	170	240	160	84.2
50	105	120	140	165	230	155	75.8
47.5	102.5	117.5	135	160	220	147.5	64.0
45	100	115	130	155	210	140	50.0
42.5	97.5	112.5	125	150	200	132.5	36.0
40	95	110	120	145	190	125	24.2
35	92.5	107.5	115	140	180	120	15.8
32.5	90	105	110	135	170	110	11.6
30	87.5	102.5	105	130	160	105	9.7
27.5	85	100	100	125	150	100	3.8
25	82.5	97.5	95	120	140	95	1.6
20	80	95	90	115	135	90	.2
17.5	77.5	92.5	85	110	130	85	.1
15	75	90	80	105	125	80	0

Body Weight Class 170–179 lbs.

Sit-Up	Curl	Upright Rowing	Over-Head Press	Bench Press	Squat	Bent-Over Rowing	%
75	124	145	185	215	315	220	100
72.5	122.5	142.5	180	210	310	212.5	99.9
70	120	140	175	205	300	205	99.8
65	117.5	137.5	170	200	290	195	99.4
62.5	115	135	165	195	280	190	98.4
60	112.5	132.5	160	190	270	182.5	96.2
57.5	110	130	155	185	260	175	90.3
55	107.5	127.5	150	180	250	165	84.2
50	105	125	145	175	240	160	75.8
47.5	102.5	122.5	140	170	235	152.5	64.0
45	100	120	135	165	225	145	50.0
42.5	97.5	117.5	130	160	215	137.5	36.0
40	95	115	125	155	205	130	24.2
35	92.5	112.5	120	150	195	125	15.8
30.5	90.5	110	115	145	185	115	11.6
30	87.5	107.5	110	140	175	110	9.7
27.5	85	105	105	135	165	105	3.8
25	82.5	102.5	100	130	155	100	1.6
20	80	100	95	125	150	95	.2
17.5	77.5	97.5	90	120	145	90	.1
15	75	95	85	115	140	85	0

Body Weight Class 180–189 lbs.

Sit-Up	Curl	Upright Rowing	Over-Head Press	Bench Press	Squat	Bent-Over Rowing	%
75	130	150	190	225	325	225	100
72.5	127.5	147.5	185	220	320	217.5	99.9
70	125	145	180	215	310	210	99.8
65	122.5	142.5	175	210	305	200	99.4
62.5	120	140	170	205	295	195	98.4
60	117.5	137.5	165	200	285	187.5	96.2
57.5	115	135	160	195	275	180	90.3
55	112.5	132.5	155	190	265	170	84.2
50	110	130	150	185	255	165	75.8
47.5	107.5	127.5	145	180	250	157.5	64.0
45	105	125	140	175	240	150	50.0
42.5	102.5	122.5	135	170	230	142.5	36.0
40	100	120	130	165	220	135	24.2
35	97.5	117.5	125	160	210	130	15.8
32.5	95	115	120	155	200	120	11.6
30	92.5	112.5	115	150	190	115	9.7
27.5	90	110	110	145	180	110	3.8
25	87.5	107.5	105	140	170	105	1.6
20	85	105	100	135	165	100	.2
17.5	82.5	102.5	95	130	155	95	.1
15	80	100	90	125	150	90	0

Body Weight Class 190 lbs.+

Sit-Up	Curl	Upright Rowing	Over-Head Press	Bench Press	Squat	Bent-Over Rowing	%
75	135	155	195	235	335	230	100
72.5	132.5	152.5	190	230	330	222.5	99.9
70	130	150	185	225	320	215	99.8
65	127.5	147.5	180	220	315	205	99.4
62.5	125	145	175	215	305	200	98.4
60	122.5	142.5	170	210	295	192.5	96.2
57.5	120	140	165	205	285	180	90.3
55	117.5	137.5	160	200	275	175	84.2
50	115	135	155	195	265	170	75.8
47.5	112.5	132.5	150	190	260	162.5	64.0
45	110	130	145	185	250	155	50.0
42.5	107.5	127.5	140	180	240	147.5	36.0
40	105	125	135	175	230	140	24.2
35	102.5	122.5	130	170	220	135	15.8
32.5	100	120	125	165	210	125	11.6
30	97.5	117.5	120	160	200	120	9.7
27.5	95	115	115	155	190	115	3.8
25	92.5	112.5	110	150	180	110	1.6
20	90	110	105	145	175	105	.2
17.5	87.5	107.5	100	140	165	100	.1
15	85	105	95	135	155	95	0

Source: Berger, R. A., *Weight Training Standards for Adult Males* (unpublished), Biokinetics Research Laboratory, Temple University, Philadelphia, PA.

appendix c

Universal Super Circuit

On the following two pages is a new high intensity program for athletes. It is designed to develop all four elements of fitness: strength, muscular endurance, cardiorespiratory endurance, and flexibility. It can be used for preseason conditioning and is a quick way to get a thorough and balanced workout.

Important Notes:

Be sure to consult your physician and obtain prior approval before engaging in this or any other strenuous training program.

Be sure to begin each exercise period by warming up and stretching to warm up the heart as well as the muscles.

The program shown on the following pages is meant to be performed on twelve Universal single-station machines, but can also be performed on a multi-station machine.

This program consists of alternating upper and lower body exercises: the aim is to reach target heart rate. See chapter 12.

Key to program: You do thirty seconds of aerobic conditioning (running in place, exercycle, jump rope etc.) between each exercise station.

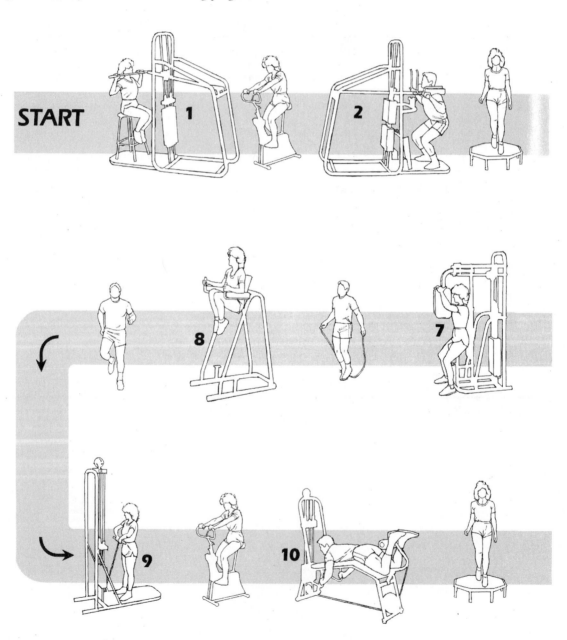

START 1 2

8 7

9 10

144

Procedures

1. How many reps? Fifteen to twenty
2. How many sets? One at each station
3. How many circuits? Three to five
4. How long at each station? Maximum thirty seconds
5. Intervals between stations. Thirty seconds of aerobic conditioning (run in place, jump rope, exercycle etc.)
6. How much weight? Forty to fifty percent maximum for average person, fifty to seventy percent for conditioned athlete
7. How to determine working weight? Find out your maximum for one lift, take percent of that for working weight. Reevaluate every six to eight weeks.

8. Breathing: Exhale as weight goes up, inhale as weight comes down.
9. Intensity: Make your muscles contract explosively throughout the full range of motion to simulate natural resistance of athletic events.
10. Cool-down: Don't head for the showers until pulse, breathing, and perspiration are back to normal. Gradually decrease body movement, reversing the way you warmed up.

At each of the numbered stations do one set of fifteen to twenty reps. Maximum thirty seconds at each station. *In between* each station, do thirty seconds of aerobic conditioning. Do the circuit three to five times.

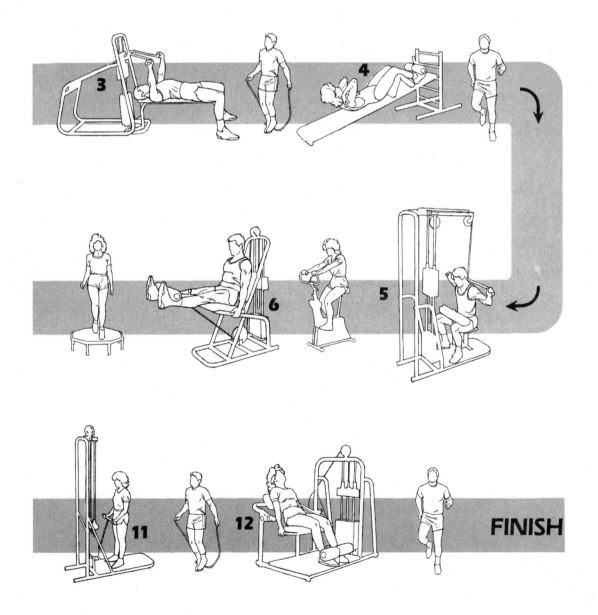

Walking/Jogging Program for Cardiorespiratory Fitness

Fitness category	Starting level
"Very poor" to "poor"	1 to 2
"Average" to "good"	2 to 3
"Very good" to "excellent"	4 to 5
"Superior"	5 to 7

Level Exercise	Heart rate training effect level (intensity)	Frequency	Duration
1 Walk for 10 to 20 minutes	60%	3 days	2 to 4 weeks
2 Walk fast for 15 to 20 minutes	60%	3 days	2 to 4 weeks
3 Jog 100 yards and then walk 300 yards. Repeat four times. Add one repetition for each succeeding exercise session. When you reach eight repetitions, move to level 4. (approximately 30 minutes)	60%	3 days	2 to 3 weeks
4 Jog 200 yards and then walk 200 yards. Repeat four times. Add one repetition for each succeeding exercise session. When you reach eight repetitions, move to level 5. (approximately 28 minutes)	60%	3 to 4 days	2 to 3 weeks
5 Jog 400 yards and then walk 400 yards. Repeat four times. Add one repetition for each succeeding exercise session. When you reach eight repetitions, move to level 6. (approximately 26 minutes)	70%	3 to 4 days	2 to 3 weeks
6 Jog 800 yards and then walk 400 yards. Repeat four times. Add one repetition for every other exercise session. When you reach six repetitions, move to level 7. (approximately 22 minutes)	70%	3 to 5 days	2 to 3 weeks

Level Exercise	Heart rate training effect level (intensity)	Frequency	Duration
7 Jog 1,200 yards and then walk 600 yards. Repeat two times. Add one repetition for every other exercise session. When you reach four repetitions, move to level 8. (approximately 22 minutes)	70%	3 to 5 days	2 to 3 weeks
8 Jog 1 mile in 10 minutes and then walk 3 minutes. Then jog 1 mile again in 10 to 12 minutes.	70%	3 to 5 days	2 to 3 weeks
9 Jog 1 1/2 miles in 15 minutes and then walk 6 to 8 minutes. Then jog again 1 1/2 miles in 15 to 18 minutes.	70%	3 to 5 days	2 to 3 weeks
10 Jog 2 miles in 20 minutes.	70%	3 to 5 days	2 to 3 weeks
11 Jog 2 miles in 18 minutes.	70%	3 to 5 days	2 to 3 weeks
12 Jog 2 miles in 16 minutes.	70%	3 to 5 days	2 to 3 weeks
13 Jog 2 miles in 14 minutes.	70%	3 to 5 days	2 to 3 weeks
14 Continue at level 13 to maintain lifetime fitness.			

Source: From *Dynamics of Fitness: A Practical Approach* by George H. McGlynn. Copyright © 1987. Wm. C. Brown Publishers, Dubuque, Iowa.

appendix e

Weight Training Progress Chart

Weight Training Record Card

Name _____

Class _____

Before

Weight	
Right Bicep	
Left Bicep	
Chest Inf.	
Chest Def.	
Abdominal Girth	
Right Thigh	
Left Thigh	
Hip	

Dates		W	R	W	R	W	R	W	R	W	R	W	R	W	R	W	R
Exercises																	
	1																
	2																
	3																
	1																
	2																
	3																
	1																
	2																
	3																
	1																
	2																
	3																
	1																
	2																
	3																
	1																
	2																
	3																
	1																
	2																
	3																

**Weight Training Record
Card**

Name _____

Class _____

After

Weight	
Right Bicep	
Left Bicep	
Chest Inf.	
Chest Def.	
Abdominal Girth	
Right Thigh	
Left Thigh	
Hip	

Dates		W	R	W	R	W	R	W	R	W	R	W	R	W	R	W	R
Exercises																	
	1																
	2																
	3																
	1																
	2																
	3																
	1																
	2																
	3																
	1																
	2																
	3																
	1																
	2																
	3																
	1																
	2																
	3																
	1																
	2																
	3																

appendix f

Sample of a Racquet Sports Mesocycle

POST SEASON

Heavy training	3 weeks
Basic strength	2 weeks
Hypertrophy	2 weeks
Basic strength	3 weeks
Active Rest	2 weeks

OFF-SEASON

Hypertrophy	2 weeks
Basic strength	5 weeks
Strength and power	3 weeks
Peaking	2 weeks
Active Rest	2 weeks
Sports Training Skills	10 weeks
Active Rest	1 week

IN-SEASON

Maintenance	8–10 weeks
Active Rest	3 weeks

appendix g

Major Vitamins and Minerals

Vitamin	Major Function	Most Reliable Sources	Deficiency	Excess (Toxicity)
A	Maintains skin and other cells that line the inside of the body; bone and tooth development; growth; vision in dim light	Liver, milk, egg yolk, deep green and yellow fruits and vegetables	Night blindness; dry skin; growth failure	Headaches, nausea, loss of hair, dry skin, diarrhea
D	Normal bone growth and development	Exposure to sunlight; fortified dairy products; eggs and fish liver oils	"Rickets" in children—defective bone formation leading to deformed bones	Appetite loss, weight loss, failure to grow
E	Prevents destruction of polyunsaturated fats caused by exposure to oxidizing agents; protects cell membranes from destruction	Vegetable oils, some in fruits and vegetables, whole grains	Breakage of red blood cells leading to anemia	Nausea and diarrhea; interferes with vitamin K if vitamin D is also deficient. Not as toxic as other fat-soluble vitamins
K	Production of blood clotting substances	Green leafy vegetables; normal bacteria that live in intestines produce K that is absorbed	Increased bleeding time	
B–1 (Thiamin)	Needed for release of energy from carbohydrates, fats, and proteins	Cereal products, pork, peas, and dried beans	Lack of energy, nerve problems	
B–2 (Riboflavin)	Energy from carbohydrates, fats, and proteins	Milk, liver, fruits and vegetables, enriched breads and cereals	Dry skin, cracked lips	
B–3 (Niacin)	Energy from carbohydrates, fats, and proteins	Liver, meat, poultry, peanut butter, legumes, enriched breads and cereals	Skin problems, diarrhea, mental depression, and eventually death (rarely occurs in U.S.)	Skin flushing, intestinal upset, nervousness, intestinal ulcers
B–6	Metabolism of protein; production of hemoglobin	White meats, whole grains, liver, egg yolk, bananas	Poor growth, anemia	Severe loss of coordination from nerve damage
B–12	Production of genetic material; maintains central nervous system	Foods of animal origin	Neurological problems, anemia	

Vitamin	Major Function	Most Reliable Sources	Deficiency	Excess (Toxicity)
Folate (Folic acid)	Production of genetic material	Wheat germ, liver, yeast, mushrooms, green leafy vegetables, fruits	Anemia	
C (Ascorbic Acid)	Formation and maintenance of connective tissue; tooth and bone formation; immune function	Fruits and vegetables	"Scurvy" (rare); swollen joints, bleeding gums, fatigue, bruising	Kidney stones, diarrhea
Pantothenic acid	Energy from carbohydrates, fats, proteins	Widely found in foods	Not observed in humans under normal conditions	
Biotin	Use of fats	Widely found in foods	Rare under normal conditions	

Minerals of Major Concern

Mineral	Major Role	Most Reliable Sources	Deficiency	Excess
Calcium	Bone and tooth formation; blood clotting; muscle contraction; nerve function	Dairy products	May lead to osteoporosis	Calcium deposits in soft tissues
Phosphorus	Skeletal development; tooth formation	Meats, dairy products, and other protein-rich foods	Rarely seen	
Sodium	Maintenance of fluid balance	Salt (sodium chloride) added to foods and sodium containing preservatives		May contribute to the development of hypertension
Iron	Formation of hemoglobin; energy from carbohydrates, fats, and proteins	Liver and red meats, enriched breads and cereals	Iron-deficiency anemia	Can cause death in children from supplement overdose
Copper	Formation of hemoglobin	Liver, nuts, shellfish, cherries, mushrooms, whole grain breads and cereals	Anemia	Nausea and vomiting
Zinc	Normal growth and development	Seafood and meats	Skin problems, delayed development, growth problems	Interferes with copper use; may decrease HDL levels
Iodine	Production of the hormone thyroxin	Iodized salt, seafood	Mental growth and retardation; lack of energy	
Fluorine	Strengthens bones and teeth	Fluoridated water	Teeth are less resistant to decay	Damage to tooth enamel

appendix h

Detailed Training Cycle for One Year (Volleyball)

1. Transitional 4 weeks

No formal or structured workouts. Activity consists of recreational sports and low-volume, low-intensity fitness activities such as swimming, jogging, tennis, basketball.

2. Preparatory Period 16–18 weeks

   a. Weeks 1 through 6

Strength Training

Mon.	3–5 sets	at	8–12 RM
Wed.	3–5 sets	at	8–12 repetitions at 75–80% of RM
Fri.	3–5 sets	at	8–12 repetitions at 75–80% of RM

Endurance   swimming, jogging, rowing, cycling etc.

| Tues. | 25–30 min. aerobic activity |
| Thurs. | 25–30 min. aerobic activity |

   b. Week 7 Unloading Week

Reduce volume and load from previous week by at least 25% in order to prepare for the next phase.

   c. Weeks 8 through 12 Strength Phase

Should participate in flexibility training before and after workout as part of warm-up and cool down.

Strength Training

Mon.	3–5 sets	5 RM
Wed.	3–5 sets	5–6 repetitions at 80–95% RM
Fri.	3–5 sets	5–6 repetitions at 80–95% RM
Tues.	20–30 min. skilled drills, sprinting, and plyometrics
Thurs.	20–30 min. skilled drills, sprinting, and plyometrics

   d. Week 13 Unloading

Reduce volume at least 25% from previous week; prepare for next phase.

   e. Week 14 through 16 Power Phase

Flexibility training same as 8th through 12th week

Strength Training

Mon.	3–5 sets	2 RM to 4 RM
Wed.	3–5 sets	2 repetitions at 70–90% of 2–4 RM
Fri.	3–5 sets	2 repetitions at 70–90% of 2–4 RM
Tues.	Practice skills
Thurs.	Practice skills

Week 17   Unloading

Recover from intense training; light activities.

Week 18   5–10% increase

Transitional Phase 2 weeks, no formal workout

Preparatory Phase

Weeks 19 through 28

19th and 20th week

Flexibility Training Before and after workout as part of warm-up and cool down.

Strength Training

Mon.	3–5 sets	8–12 repetitions at 70% of 1 RM
Wed.	3–5 sets	8–12 repetitions at 60% of 1 RM
Fri.	3–5 sets	8–12 repetitions at 50% of 1 RM

Weeks 21 through 22

Mon.	3–5 sets	8–12 repetitions at 85% of 1 RM
Wed.	3–5 sets	8–12 repetitions at 80% of 1 RM
Fri.	3–5 sets	8–12 repetitions at 70% of 1 RM
Tues.	20–25 min. anaerobic or aerobics depending on activity	
Thurs.	20–25 min. anaerobic or aerobics depending on activity	

Week 23   Unloading

Strength Training

Mon.	1–3 sets	2–4 repetitions at 80% of 1 RM
Wed.	1–3 sets	2–4 repetitions at 70% of 1 RM
Fri.	1–3 sets	2–4 repetitions at 60% of 1 RM

Week 24 through 27

Mon.	3–5 sets	2–4 repetitions at 95% of 1 RM
Wed.	3–5 sets	2–4 repetitions at 80% of 1 RM
Fri.	3–5 sets	2–4 repetitions at 70% of 1 RM

Week 28

Mon.	1–2 sets	1 RM
Wed.	1–2 sets	1 RM
Fri.	1–2 sets	1 repetition at 70% of 1 RM

Pre-Season

Transition Weeks 29 through 30

Preparatory Phase   Weeks 31 through 37

Week 31 through 32

Mon.	1–3 sets	8–10 repetitions at 70% of 1 RM
Thurs.	1–3 sets	8–10 repetitions at 75% of 1 RM

Week 33

Mon.	1–3 sets	5–6 repetitions at 85% of 1 RM
Thurs.	1–3 sets	5–6 repetitions at 80% of 1 RM

Week 34

Mon.	1–3 sets	2–4 repetitions at 90% of 1 RM
Thurs.	1–3 sets	2–4 repetitions at 80% of 1 RM

Week 35

Mon.	1–3 sets	2–4 repetitions at 95% of 1 RM
Thurs.	1–3 sets	2–4 repetitions at 80% of 1 RM

Week 36

Mon.	1–3 sets	1 RM
Thurs.	1–3 sets	1 RM

Competition

Week 37 to End of Competition

Week 37

1 set	10 repetitions at 75% of 1 RM

Week 38

1 set	5–6 repetitions at 80% of 1 RM

Week 39

1 set	5–6 repetitions at 85% of 1 RM

Week 40

1 set	2–4 repetitions at 90% of 1 RM

Week 41

| 1 set | 2–4 repetitions at 95% of 1 RM |

Week 42

| 1 set | 2–4 repetitions at 95% of 1 RM |

Week 43

| 1 set | 2–4 repetitions at 95% of 1 RM |

Week 44

| 1 set | 2–4 repetitions at 95% of 1 RM |

Week 45

| 1 set | 2–4 repetitions at 100% of 1 RM |

Adapted from Dan Wathen, Periodization, concepts and applications, in *Essentials of Strength Training and Conditioning,* ed. Thomas R. Baechle. (Champaign, IL: Human Kinetics, 1994).

appendix i

Suggested Readings

Motivation

Garfield, Charles A., and Hal Z. Bennett. 1984. *Peak Performance—Mental Training Techniques of the World's Greatest Athletes.* Los Angeles, CA: J. P. Tharcher.

Jerome, John. 1984. *Staying With It.* New York: The Viking Press.

Suinn, R. M. 1980. *Psychology in Sports: Methods and Applications.* Minneapolis, MN: Burgess.

Tutko, Thomas A., and Umberto Tosi. 1976. *Sports Psyching—Playing Your Best Game All of the Time.* Los Angeles, CA: J. P. Tharcher.

Williams, Jean M. 1986. *Applied Sports Psychology.* Palo Alto, CA.: Mayfield Press.

Nutrition and Weight Control

Briggs, George M., and Doris H. Calloway. 1979. *Bogert's Nutrition and Physical Fitness.* Philadelphia: Saunders.

Brody, Jane. 1981. *Jane Brody's Nutrition Book.* New York: Norton.

Guthrie, Helen. 1983. *Introductory Nutrition.* St. Louis: C. V. Mosby.

Katch, Frank I., and William D. McArdle. 1977. *Nutrition, Weight Control and Exercise.* Boston: Houghton Mifflin.

Whitney, Eleanor N., and Corinne B. Bataldo. 1983. *Understanding Normal and Clinical Nutrition.* St. Paul: West.

Wardlaw, Gordon, Paul M. Insel, and Marcia Sexler. 1994. *Contemporary, Issues and Insights.* St. Louis: Mosby.

Physical Fitness and Health

Allsen, Phillip E., Joyce M. Harrison, and Barbara Vance. 1984. *Fitness for Life,* 3d ed. Dubuque, IA: Wm. C. Brown Publishers.

Cooper, Kenneth. 1982. *Aerobics Program for Total Well Being.* New York: Evans.

Corbin, Charles, and Ruth Lindsey. 1985. *Concepts of Physical Fitness with Laboratories.* 5th ed. Dubuque, IA: Wm. C. Brown Publishers.

Di Gennaro, Joseph. 1983. *The New Physical Fitness: Exercise for Every Body.* Englewood, CO: Morton.

Dintiman, George B., Stephan E. Stone, Jude C. Pennington, and Robert G. Davis. 1984. *Discovering Lifetime Fitness.* St. Paul, MN: West.

Falls, Arnold B., Ann M. Baylor, and Rud K. Dishman. 1980. *Essentials of Fitness.* Philadelphia: Saunders.

Getchell, Bud. 1983. *Physical Fitness, A Way of Life.* 3d. ed. New York: Wiley.

Marley, William. 1982. *Health and Physical Fitness.* Philadelphia: Saunders.

McGlynn, George H. 1987. *Dynamics of Fitness/A Practical Approach.* Dubuque, IA: Wm. C. Brown Publishers.

Pollock, Michael, Jack H. Wilmore, and Samuel M. Fox. 1984. *Exercise in Health and Disease.* Philadelphia: Saunders.

Prentice, William. 1994. *Fitness for College and Life.* 4th ed. St. Louis: Mosby.

Rosensweig, S. 1982. *Sports Fitness for Women.* New York: Harper & Row.

Wilmore, Jack. 1986. *Sensible Fitness.* Leisure Press.

Physiology of Exercise

Brooks, George A., and Thomas D. Fahey. 1984. *Exercise Physiology.* New York: John Wiley & Sons.

DeVries, Herbert A. 1980. *Physiology of Exercise for Physical Education and Athletics.* 3d ed. Philadelphia: Saunders.

Fox, E. L. 1979. *Sports Physiology.* Philadelphia: Saunders.

Fox, Edward, Richard Bowers, and Merle Foss. 1993. *The Physiological Basis for Exercise and Sport.* 5th ed. Dubuque, IA: Brown & Benchmark.

Lamb, David R. 1984. *Physiology of Exercise.* New York: Macmillan.

Powers, Scott K., and Edward T. Howley. 1994. *Exercise Physiology.* 2d ed. Dubuque, IA: Brown & Benchmark.

Shaver, Larry G. 1981. *Essentials of Exercise Physiology.* Minneapolis: Burgess.

Wilmore, Jack H. 1982. *Training for Sport and Activity, The Physiological Basis of Conditioning.* 2d ed. Boston: Allyn & Bacon.

Wells, C. L. 1985. *Women, Sport and Performance, A Physiological Perspective.* Champaign, IL: Human Kinetics Publisher.

Strength and Muscle Development

Bass, Charles. 1980. *Ripped—The Sensible Way to Achieve Ultimate Muscularity.* Albuquerque, NM.: Ripped Enterprises.

Darden, Ellington. 1982. *The Nautilus Book.* Chicago: Contemporary Books.

Darden, Ellington. 1983. *The Nautilus Woman.* New York: Simon & Schuster.

Essentials of Strength Training and Conditioning. 1994. Ed. Thomas Baechle. Champaign, IL: Human Kinetics.

Fleck, Steven S., and William Kraemer. 1987. *Designing Resistance Training Programs.* Champaign, IL: Human Kinetics.

Fox, E. L., and D. K. Mathews. 1974. *Interval Training, Conditioning for Sport and General Fitness.* Philadelphia: Saunders.

Gaines, Charles, and George Butler. 1984. *Pumping Iron II: The Unprecedented Woman.* New York: Simon & Schuster.

Hatfield, Frederick C. *The Complete Guide To Power Training.* New Orleans. Fitness Systems, 1983, Lakewood, CA: Sports Conditioning Services, 5542 South Street, 90713.

Jarrell, Steve. 1982. *Working Out with Weights.* New York: Anco.

Kennedy, Robert. 1985. *Reps!—Building Massive Muscle!* New York: Sterling Publishing Co.

Kirkley, George W. 1982. *Weight Lifting and Weight Training*. New York: Anco.

Lance, Kathryn. 1978. *Getting Strong—A Woman's Guide to Realizing Her Physical Potential*. New York: The Bobbs-Merrill Co.

Leon, Edie. 1976. *Complete Woman Weight Training Guide*. Mountain View, CA: Anderson World.

Lyon, Lisa, and Douglas Kent Hall. 1981. *Lisa Lyon's Body Magic*. New York: Bantam Books.

O'Shea, J. P. 1979. *Scientific Principles and Methods of Strength Fitness*. Reading, MA: Addison-Wesley.

Pearl, Bill, and Gary Moran. 1986. *Getting Stronger*. Bolinas, CA: Shelter.

Perrin, David H. 1993. *Isokinetic Exercise and Assessment*. Champaign, IL: Human Kinetics.

Pirie, Lynne, and Bill Reynolds. 1984. *Getting Built—A Woman's Body Building Program for Strength, Beauty and Fitness*. New York: Warner Books.

Sobey, Edwin. 1981. *Strength Training Book*. Mountain View, CA: Anderson World.

Stone, M., and H. O'Bryant. *Weight Training: A Scientific Approach*. Minneapolis, MN: Burgess.

Strength and Power in Sport. 1993. Ed. P. U. Komi. Blackwell.

Todd, Jan, and Terry Todd. 1985. *Lift Your Way to Youthful Fitness—The Comprehensive Guide to Weight Training*. Boston: Little Brown & Co.

Webster, David. 1979. *Body Building—An Illustrated History*. New York: Arco Publishing, Inc.

Westcott, Wayne. 1983. *Strength Fitness Physiological Principles and Training Techniques*. Boston: Allyn & Bacon.

Wright, James E. 1978. *Anabolic Steroids and Sports*. Natick, MA: Sports Science Consultants.

credits

Photographs

George H. McGlynn and Gary T. Moran

Photo Reproduction

Agfa Gevaert

Models

Barbara Gaenslen, George C. McGlynn, Pernella Alser,
and Bacari Harris

Locations

Mariner Square Athletic Club
Alameda, CA
University of San Francisco
San Francisco, CA

Index

Cardiorespiratory training
   aerobic running program for, 146–147
   aerobic versus anaerobic exercises, 92
   benefits of, 92
   cautions about, 98–99
   circuit training, 96
   cool down, 96
   and duration, 94–95
   exercise prescription, 97
   and frequency, 95–96
   heart rate, determination of, 93
   and intensity, 93
   screening, pre-exercise, 96–97
Carnitine, 128
Cheating, in weight training program, 21–22, 58
Childbirth, exercise after, 89
Chin-ups, 57
Chromium, 128
Chronic hypertrophy, 51
Circuit training
   example program, 98
   nature of, 96
   universal super circuit program, 144–145
Cocaine, 128, 129
Compression, for injuries, 114
Concentration, meaning of, 30, 32
Conditioning, definition of, 5
Contract-relax stretching method, 102
Cool down, 96, 99
Cortisone, for injuries, 114
Cross-country skiing machine, 134
Crunches, 78
Cybex knee extension, 132
Cybex 600, 132

D

Dead lift, 20
Declined bench press, 70
Deltoids, 48, 49
   exercises for, 53, 73–74
Desiccated organs, 128
Diets
   evaluation of, 119–120
   fad diets, 122
   Food Guide Pyramid, 120, 121
   fraudulent, 120
   information sources on, 157

protein-supplemented diets, 120, 122
   vitamin-supplemented diets, 122
Dislocation, nature of, 113, 115
Diuretic, 129
Drugs
   amphetamines, 127
   anabolic steroids, 125–127
   beta-adrenergic agonists, 128
   caffeine, 127
   carnitine, 128
   chromium/vanadium, 128
   cocaine, 128
   erythropoietin, 128
   growth hormones, 127
   steroid replacers, 128
Drug testing, 126
Duration
   and cardiovascular fitness, 94–95
   definition of, 14, 22, 99
Dynamic flexibility, 8–9

E

Eccentric loading
   advantages/disadvantages of, 59
   nature of, 57, 60
Elevation, for injuries, 114
Endurance
   cardiovascular, 8, 10
   definition of, 8
   muscle, 5, 8
   and sports activities, 8
Energy
   and ATP, 48, 93, 119
   expended during exercise, 119
   sources during exercise, 93
Epimysium, 47, 49, 53
Equipment
   CAM II, 132
   categories of, 131
   free weights, 131, 133
   Hydra fitness, 133
   isokinetic machines, 132
   Nautilus, 132
   Polaris, 133
   power exercise equipment, 133–134
   resistance machines, 131
   universal machine, 132
Erector spinae, exercises for, 53, 80
Erythropoietin, 128
Exercise physiology, information sources on, 157
Extensor digitorum communis, 48

F

Fad diets, 122
Fast-twitch fibers, nature of, 51, 53
Fats, 123
   nutritional requirements, 118
Fitness
   and body composition, 9
   and cardiorespiratory endurance, 8
   and endurance, 8
   and flexibility, 8–9
   and muscle power, 9
   and strength, 7
Flexibility
   activities for, 9
   assessment of, 38
   definition of, 8, 10, 46, 101, 109
   dynamic, 8-9
   physiological factors, 101
   and range of motion, 19, 102
   and resistance training, 101
   static, 9
   See also Stretching
Flexor carpi radialis, 48
   exercises for, 53, 77
Flexor carpi ulnaris, exercises for, 77
Food Guide Pyramid, 120, 121
Forced repetition, nature of, 62, 67
Forearm curls, 77
Forearm extensors, 48
Forearm flexors, 49
   exercises for, 77
Fractures, nature of, 113
Free weights, 57, 131, 133
Frequency
   and cardiovascular training, 95–96
   definition of, 14, 22, 99

G

Gastrocnemius, 48, 49
   exercises for, 53, 85
Gloves, benefits of use, 21
Gluteus maximus, 49
   exercises for, 53, 81–82
Gluteus medius, 48, 49
   exercises for, 83
Glycogen, as energy source, 93
Goal setting, 28–29
Gracilus, 49
Growth hormones, 127